23

Recent Advances in
Anaesthesia and Intensive Care

This is the latest volume of this very successful and long-established series (previously entitled *Recent Advances in Anaesthesia and Analgesia*) to present a collection of cutting-edge topics for anaesthetists. It has been complied by some of the world's leading authorities in their subjects and builds on the successful formula of the previous volumes. As the title suggests, these latest volumes have increased the input from the field of intensive care, and the emphasis remains on producing articles of high quality and interest to the reader while providing exceptional value for money.

This volume is a recommended reading for trainee, practising anaesthetists and intensivists at all levels of experience.

23

Recent Advances in
Anaesthesia and Intensive Care

Edited by

J.N. Cashman BSc, MB BS, BA, MD, FRCA
Consultant Anaesthetist, St George's Hospital, London
Honorary Senior Lecturer in Anaesthesia
University of London, UK

R.M. Grounds MB BS, MRCS LRCP, MD, FRCA, DA
Consultant in Anaesthesia and Intensive Care Medicine
St George's Hospital, London
Honorary Reader in Intensive Care Medicine
University of London, UK

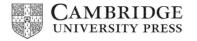

CAMBRIDGE
UNIVERSITY PRESS

PUBLISHED BY THE PRESS SYNDICATE OF THE UNIVERSITY OF CAMBRIDGE
The Pitt Building, Trumpington Street, Cambridge, United Kingdom

CAMBRIDGE UNIVERSITY PRESS
The Edinburgh Building, Cambridge CB2 2RU, UK
40 West 20th Street, New York, NY 10011-4211, USA
477 Williamstown Road, Port Melbourne, VIC 3207, Australia
Ruiz de Alarcón 13, 28014 Madrid, Spain
Dock House, The Waterfront, Cape Town 8001, South Africa

http://www.cambridge.org

First published 2005

Printed in the United Kingdom at the University Press, Cambridge

Typeface: Sabon 10.5/13pt   System: QuarkXpress®

A catalog record for this book is available from the British Library

ISBN 1 841 10 145 1

The publisher has used its best endeavors to ensure that the URLs
for external websites referred to in this book are correct and
active at the time of going to press. However, the publisher has
no responsibility for the websites and can make no guarantee
that a site will remain live or that the content is or will
remain appropriate.

Every effort has been made in preparing this book to provide accurate
and up-to-date information that is in accord with accepted standards
and practice at the time of publication. Nevertheless, the authors,
editors and publisher can make no warranties that the information
contained herein is totally free from error, not least because clinical
standards are constantly changing through research and regulation.
The authors, editors and publisher therefore disclaim all liability for
direct or consequential damages resulting from the use of material
contained in this book. Readers are strongly advised to pay careful
attention to information provided by the manufacturer of any drugs
or equipment that they plan to use.

Contents

Preface

In this 23rd edition of *Recent Advances in Anaesthesia and Intensive Care*, we bid farewell to our Senior Co-editor Prof. Anthony (Tony) Adams. Tony joined Dr Richard Atkinson for the 15th edition, which appeared in 1985 and has been a co-editor of *Recent Advances* through eight editions over the past 20 years. When Dr Atkinson stepped down as editor, Tony invited Dr Jeremy Cashman to co-edit the 19th edition. Dr Michael Grounds joined the editorial team for the 22nd edition. Tony's drive, enthusiasm and wisdom born of long experience have been in no small measure instrumental in the continuing popularity of the series. Both of the current editors are grateful to Tony for his wise counsel over the years and for his continuing support, even now when he is no longer an editor. We wish him a long, healthy and happy retirement.

The editors are grateful to the many distinguished colleagues from the USA, Europe and the UK who have contributed to this volume. We have endeavoured to include a range of topics in this issue that represent all aspects of anaesthesia and intensive care. The first four chapters present developments in the basic sciences. There is enormous inter-individual variability in the way patients respond to medications. Indeed, adapting to this heterogeneity is part of the 'art' of anaesthesia. Over recent years, huge progress has been made in our understanding of the structure as well as the function of the genome, allowing researchers to explore those genes that express proteins controlling drug action and metabolism. The burgeoning field of pharmacogenomics deals with the various aspects of gene–drug interactions and aims to further elucidate the inherited nature of inter-individual differences in drug disposition and effects. In Chapter 1 *Pharmacogenomics: the genetic basis for variability in drug response*, Dr Sweeney reviews the current status of work in this field, highlights anaesthetic examples and addresses strategies that hold promise for the future; recombinant DNA technology has already resulted in the introduction of drugs, such as recombinant human activated protein C (Chapter 8) and human insulin (Chapter 9). In Chapter 2 *The opioid receptor and opioid peptides*, Dr Zöllner and Prof. Stein review recent developments in the understanding of opioid receptors. Molecular cloning has had a tremendous impact on our knowledge of the μ-, δ- and κ-opioid receptors, as well as identifying the opioid-like orphan receptor 1 (ORL-1). Cellular mechanisms of action including opioid receptor desensitization (important in the development of tolerance; Chapter 10) and endogenous ligands are discussed. The functional aspects of opioid use with specific reference to their peripheral antinociceptive effect are considered. Normal haemostasis is achieved by a complex mechanism comprising a balance between pro- and anti-coagulant forces. Hereditary or acquired deficiency of factors on either side of this balance may result in a prothrombotic or a haemorrhagic tendency. The system is continually active at a low rate, which allows it to be rapidly responsive to haemorrhagic challenge. Separation of the physiological trigger for coagulation from the effector enzymes in plasma is essential for controlling this system. In Chapter 3 *Coagulation*, Dr Laffan explains how improved understanding allows us to effectively manipulate this system and treat these disorders for therapeutic benefit. It has become apparent that anaesthetic drugs can influence the heart by augmenting or inhibiting (or indeed having no overall effect) on cardioprotective mechanisms. Prof. Schlack and Dr Ebel, in Chapter 4 *Anaesthetic agents and myocardial protection*, point out the evidence that cardioprotection by anaesthetic agents can be elicited in the clinical setting and may add to other organ protection strategies. Volatile anaesthetic agents can interfere with ischaemic preconditioning, may act against reperfusion injury and as a result may impact on patient outcome in ischaemia–reperfusion situations.

The next two chapters deal with trauma and emergency medicine topics. As Drs Gardner and McDonagh state in Chapter 5 *The treatment of heart failure due to left ventricular systolic dysfunction*, heart failure is a serious condition, with a worse prognosis than many forms of cancer, that affects a significant proportion of the population. Until recently, the goal for the treatment of heart failure was to relieve symptoms and enhance functional capacity. However, recent studies have shown that pharmacotherapy with angiotensin converting enzyme inhibitors and β-adrenergic receptor blockade and cardiac resynchronization therapy combined with automatic implantable cardioverter defibrillator implantation can reduce both the morbidity and the mortality of chronic heart failure. Drs Gardner and McDonagh also present the results of recent trials of nesiritide and levosimendan in acute heart failure. Blunt chest trauma remains an extreme clinical challenge, accounting for nearly 25% of all traumatic deaths. Life-threatening chest lesions are frequently associated with extrathoracic injuries that may contribute to severe, sometimes delayed, cardio-respiratory failure. However, apparently minor trauma may also be life threatening. In Chapter 6 *Blunt chest trauma*, Drs Edouard, Minville and Martin present the management of this condition, including the use of new imaging technology in the assessment of trauma patients. A specific, step-wise therapeutic strategy is outlined.

Two of the primary goals of haemodynamic monitoring are to identify the presence of circulatory shock and to guide specific goal-directed treatments. In Chapter 7 *Functional haemodynamic monitoring* Drs Chavko and Pinsky present recent advances in monitoring techniques and review clinical trials that support the rationale of applying 'functional' measures of cardiovascular performance to define specific treatment approaches, rather than just the measurement of static haemodynamic values that may reflect a variety of disease processes and their potential responsiveness to treatments. The limitations of the technique are also presented.

The next three chapters consider intensive care topics. Sepsis is one of the most common disease processes encountered in the critically ill population. Sepsis has been, and continues to be, the subject of vast amounts of research, and sepsis therapeutics in particular is a rapidly advancing field. In Chapter 8 *Sepsis and the use of Xigris®*, Prof. Vincent reviews drotrecogin alfa, a recombinant form of the natural protein activated protein C (Xigris®). Xigris is the first immunomodulating drug to be shown to directly influence outcome in patients with severe sepsis and septic shock. The next chapter presents another approach to the problem of infection, acquired either before or after admission to the intensive care unit (ICU). The purpose of selective decontamination of the digestive tract is to prevent or eradicate oropharyngeal and gastrointestinal carriage of potentially pathogenic micro-organisms, leaving the indigenous flora predominantly undisturbed. In Chapter 9 *Selective decontamination of the digestive tract: why don't we apply evidence in practice?* Drs van Saene, Taylor, Barrett, Lowry and Sarginson review the evidence in favour of selective decontamination and propose a radical rethinking of the philosophy by which antimicrobials are used. In the past, hyperglycaemia was considered to be an adaptive stress response, and a rise in blood sugar in critical illness was only treated when blood glucose levels became excessive. However, a recent study clearly established the beneficial effects of strictly maintaining normoglycaemia in ICU patients. Intensive insulin therapy was associated with a remarkable reduction in mortality of ICU patients, particularly in patients with prolonged critical illness. In Chapter 10 *Glycaemic control and outcome in intensive care*, Drs Mesotten, Vanhorebeek and Van den Berghe discuss the mechanisms for this action and describe a regimen for maintaining strict glycaemic control.

Anaesthesia and postoperative analgesia in patients dependent on psychoactive substances poses special problems. These patients commonly suffer from co-existent medical and psychiatric illness. In Chapter 11 *Substance use disorders and anaesthesia*, Prof. Jage introduces the concept of substance use disorders with central nervous system depressant and stimulant substances. The neural basis of addiction is described and the anaesthetic and analgesic management of patients with substance use disorders and ex-addicts is outlined in detail.

This edition of Recent Advances aims to afford practising anaesthetists the opportunity to keep abreast of some of the latest developments in our speciality. In addition, the editors feel that it is important that the present volume addresses the whole scope of our speciality from the laboratory to the operating theatre. We hope that readers not only find the chapters in this issue stimulating and interesting but also agree with this approach.

London   J.N.C.
July 2004   R.M.G.

Contributors

Dr S.P. Barrett
Department of Bacteriology
Charing Cross Hospital
Fulham Palace Road
London, W6 8RF
UK

Prof. Greet Van den Berghe
Professor and Head of Department of Intensive Care Medicine
University Hospital Gasthuisberg
University of Leuven
B-3000 Leuven
Belgium

Dr R. Chavko
University of Pittsburgh School of Medicine
606 Scaife Hall
3550 Terrace Street
Pittsburgh, PA 15261
USA

Dr D. Ebel
Klinik fur Anaesthesiologie
Universitastklinikum Dusseldorf
Moorenstrasse 5
40225 Dusseldorf
Germany

Dr A. Edouard
Service d'Anesthésie-Réanimation
Centre Hospitalier de Bicêtre
94275 Le Kremlin Bicêtre
France

Dr R.S. Gardner
Department of Medical Cardiology
University of Glasgow
Glasgow Royal Infirmary
10 Alexandra Parade
Glasgow G31 2ER
UK

Prof. Dr Jurgen Jage
Director of Pain Services
Klinik fur Anaesthesiologie
University Hospital Mainz
Langenbeckstrasse 1, 5513
Mainz
Germany

Dr Michael Laffan
Department of Haematology
Faculty of Medicine, 4th Floor Commonwealth Building
Imperial College School of Medicine
Hammersmith Hospital
Du Cane Road
London W12 0NN
UK

Dr K. Lowry
Consultant in Intensive Care Medicine
Department of Intensive Care
Royal Victoria Hospital
Grosvenor Road
Belfast, BT12 6BA
Northern Ireland
UK

Dr L. Martin
Service d'Anesthésie-Réanimation
Centre Hospitalier de Bicêtre
94275 Le Kremlin Bicêtre
France

Dr Theresa McDonagh
Department of Medical Cardiology
University of Glasgow
Glasgow Royal Infirmary
10 Alexandra Parade
Glasgow G31 2ER
UK

Dr D. Mesotten
Department of Intensive Care Medicine
University Hospital Gasthuisberg
University of Leuven
B-3000 Leuven
Belgium

Dr V. Minville
Service d'Anesthésic-Réanimation
Centre Hospitalier de Bicêtre
94275 Le Kremlin Bicêtre
France

Prof. Michael R. Pinsky
University of Pittsburgh School of Medicine
606 Scaife Hall
3550 Terrace Street
Pittsburgh, PA 15261
USA

Dr H.K.F. van Saene
Consultant/Reader in Medical Microbiology
Department of Medical Microbiology
University of Liverpool
Duncan Building
Daulby Street
Liverpool L69 3GA
UK

Dr R.E. Sarginson
Department of Anaesthesia and Intensive Care
Royal Liverpool Children's Hospital Alder Hey
Eaton Road, West Derby
Liverpool
Merseyside L12 2AP
UK

Prof. Dr Wolfgang Schlack
Leitender Oberarzt
Klinik fur Anaesthesiologie
Universitastklinikum Dusseldorf
Moorenstrasse 5
40225 Dusseldorf
Germany

Prof. Dr C. Stein
Direktor, Klinik für Anaesthesiologie
Campus Benjamin Franklin
Freie Universität Berlin
Hindenburgdamm 30
D-12200 Berlin
Germany

Dr B. Sweeney
Department of Anaesthesia
Royal Bournemouth Hospital
Castle Lane East
Bournemouth
Dorset BH7 7DW
UK

Dr N. Taylor
Department of Medical Microbiology
University of Liverpool
Duncan Building
Daulby Street
Liverpool L69 3GA
UK

Dr I. Vanhorebeek
Department of Intensive Care Medicine
University Hospital Gasthuisberg
University of Leuven
B-3000 Leuven
Belgium

Prof. Jean-Louis Vincent
Head, Department of Intensive Care
Erasme Hospital
Route de Lennick 808
B-1070 Brussels
Belgium

Dr C. Zöllner
Klinik für Anaesthesiologie
Campus Benjamin Franklin
Freie Universität Berlin
Hindenburgdamm 30
D-12200 Berlin
German

B.P. Sweeney

Pharmacogenomics: the genetic basis for variability in drug response

"If it were not for the great variability among individuals, medicine might as well be a science and not an art."

Sir William Osler, 1892

Since the unravelling of the structure of DNA by Watson and Crick half a century ago, the scientific community has plunged into a headlong quest to unlock the secrets of the human genome which culminated in the recent successful completion of the Human Genome Project (HGP).[1] Among the surprises which accompanied the completion of this gargantuan task, were the relative paucity of genes identified in comparison with other species (a mere 32,000 compared with 19,000 of the tiny nematode *Caenorhabditis elegans*),[2] secondly, the extent of redundant or non-coding sequences some-times referred to as 'junk' *DNA*, and thirdly the relative lack of variation between individuals or among racial groups. More surprising perhaps, is the similarity between *Homo sapiens* and other species. For example, the genome of man and the chimpanzee are 98.8% identical,[3] 75% of the dog's genome is shared with man[4] and even lower life forms have sizeable lengths of DNA which are identical to areas in the human genome. Other findings which have intrigued investigators are the widespread occurrence of duplicated non-functioning genes, so-called 'pseudogenes', and the presence of evidence of contamination of the genome by retroviruses, similar to the human immunodeficiency virus (HIV) that causes AIDS. Given that 98% of the genome represents a *terra incognita* for the gene explorer and that a function can be ascribed to only half of those genes already discovered, the huge breakthroughs already accomplished represent but a small step in genome-based science. Nevertheless, as technology provides ever more sophisticated tools for scientific investigation, so too do the secrets of human biodiversity unfold. For example, the central dogma of 'one gene, one transcript, one protein' is now no longer viable. A single gene may encrypt, by a process of differential splicing, several transcripts and therefore, potentially many different proteins, thus elucidating the apparent imbalance between the size of the genome and the 100,000 or so proteins which comprise the proteome.

Physicians have long been aware of illness caused by single-gene abnormalities. However, greater understanding of the structure as well as the function of the genome is casting new light on the aetiology of diverse conditions such as hypertension, asthma, thromboembolic disease, diabetes and schizophrenia and allowing researchers to explore new and exciting avenues of therapy. One particular area of genomics which has already revolutionized drug research and whose clinical relevance continues to grow, is the study of those genes that express proteins controlling drug action and metabolism. Perhaps more importantly, as the genome divulges its secrets, those genes which are putatively associated with disease, that is *candidate genes*, together with their respective products, will increasingly be the focus of attention of pharmaceutical companies and these will thereby become the new drug targets. Until recently, the term pharmacogenetics was used to describe, in simple Mendelian terms, the influence of single genes on drug action. The exponential growth of genomic science has inevitably led to a re-evaluation of genetically determined responses to medications and has necessitated the creation of a new discipline, termed 'pharmacogenomics', which deals with the various aspects of gene–drug interactions including not only the effects of altered drug disposition as a result of altered metabolism, but also interesting effects resulting from mutations in receptors, transporters and biosynthetic pathways. The parallel development in information technology has given birth to new disciplines such as computer-based gene discovery ('bioinformatics'), and the development of automated, miniaturized techniques has permitted the development of new and exciting ways of studying gene expression. This in turn has facilitated new understanding of disease and its treatment. Although at present the impact of these new discoveries has been modest, the tempo of discovery is quickening and soon genomic science will impact every facet of medicine including anaesthesia and intensive care.

History of Pharmacogenetics

All anaesthetists are aware of the inherited abnormality of succinylcholine metabolism, which results from a deficiency in plasma cholinesterase activity leading to prolonged paralysis, a condition present in approximately 1:3500 of the population. This varied response of patients to succinylcholine was elucidated in the 1950s by Kalow[5] and was one of the first examples of inherited differences in drug metabolism to be recognized in modern times. Although the earliest recorded evidence of individual difference in metabolism can be traced back to classical times, the discipline of 'pharmacogenetics' emerged first of all from knowledge acquired by scientists such as Mendel,[6] the father of genetics, who set out the laws of inherited characteristics which now bear his name. Subsequently, our understanding of biochemical genetics was improved by the English physician Achibald Garrod, who coined the term 'inborn error of metabolism', detecting individual abnormalities of intermediary metabolism resulting from mutations in genes controlling enzyme synthesis.[7] Subsequently, Snyder discovered that the sense of taste was subject to genetic variability.[8]

The first idiosyncratic reaction to a foreign substance, or xenobiotic, is said to have been recognized by the ancient Greeks who noted that some individuals who consumed fava beans, a staple diet in the region, were prone to haematuria. It is now known that the reason for this phenomenon is a deficiency of the enzyme glucose 6-phosphate dehydrogenase (G-6 PD), a condition particularly prevalent among Caucasians of Mediterranean origin, affecting around 100 million people worldwide and as well as around 14% of American Negroes. During World War II many black American soldiers who served in areas of the globe where malaria was endemic received the antimalarial drug primaquine, which unfortunately can also induce haemolysis in G-6 PD deficient individuals. A significant number of these soldiers developed haematuria as a result.[9] After World War II, medicine entered the era of antibiotics. This heralded the treatment of serious and potentially lethal infections such as tuberculosis. One of the first antibiotics to be introduced was isoniazid. Shortly after its introduction however, it was noted that some patients developed peripheral neuropathy. Investigation revealed that this toxicity resulted from high blood concentrations of the drug as a result of impaired activity of the enzyme N-acetyltransferase (NAT).[10] These patients were labelled 'slow-acetylators'. The recognition of these genetically determined differences in drug metabolism in the post-war years attracted the attention of researchers, such as Motulsky,[11] and Kalow[12] who wrote the first comprehensive textbook on heredity and the response to drugs. The work of these scientists laid the foundations for the discipline of 'pharmacogenetics', a term coined in 1959 by Friedrich Vogel.[13]

Significant milestones in pharmacogenetics were the recognition in the 1970s of abnormalities in the breakdown of the hypotensive drug debrisoquine by the enzyme debrisoquine hydroxylase (later termed

Table 1.1 Some important milestones in the history of pharmacogenomics

Date	Author	Discovery	Reference
1866	Mendel	Lays down the principles of heredity	6
1909	Garrod	Publication of 'Inborn Errors of Metabolism'	7
1932	Snyder	Characterization of the *phenylthiourea-non-taster* as an autosomal recessive trait	8
1954	Hughes *et al.*	Relates isoniazid neuropathy to metabolism	10
1956	Carson *et al.*	Discovery of glucose G-6 PD deficiency	9
1957	Kalow	Characterizes acetylcholinesterase deficiency	5
1957	Motulsky	Explanation for the inherited differences in drug metabolism	11
1957	Vogel	Coins the term 'pharmakogenetik'	13
1960	Price Evans	Characterization of acetylators polymorphisms	
1962	Kalow	The first textbook on pharmacogenetics	12
1977	Mahgoub *et al.*	Description of the debrisoquine polymorphism	14
1979	Eichelbaum *et al.*	Describes sparteine metabolism polymorphism	28
1980	Weinshilboum & Sladek	Description of genetics of mercaptopurine metabolism	15
1982	Eichelbaum *et al.*	Recognition of link between sparteine and debrisoquine metabolism	29
1984	Wedlund *et al.*	Description of the cytochrome CYP2C19 polymorphism	16
1988	Gonzalez	Explanation for the debrisoquine phenotype	30
1992	Grant & Meyer	Explanation of the molecular genetics of NAT	64
1997	Yates *et al.*	Polymerase chain reaction (PCR) based methods used to detect thiopurine *S*-methyl transferase (TPMT) deficiency	58

CYP2D6),[14] and the recognition of thiopurine S-methyl transferase (TPMT) deficiency among leukaemic patients, as an explanation for the sometimes lethal complication arising from mercaptopurine and azathioprine therapy.[15] Further polymorphisms relating to other cytochrome (CYP) enzymes were discovered in the subsequent decade (Table 1.1).[16]

The source of interindividual variability

There are two main types of interindividual variation which have been found in the genome. The first is a variation in the number of recurring small sequences (micro-satellites) which occur among the non-coding 'junk' DNA and which are known as 'variable number tandem repeats' (VNTRs). These are commonly used, particularly in forensic pathology, as a means of DNA fingerprinting and in paternity testing. The second and most important source of variation in the genome is the single nucleotide polymorphism (SNP or snip). A consortium set up in 1999 to chart the extent of these differences found 1.4 million SNPs among the 3 billion or so base pairs which comprise the genome (only 1% of these, however, are in exonic, i.e. coding, sequences).[17] New SNPs are continually being discovered and currently the estimated total number is around 3 million. In other words, there is only a 0.08% difference between members of the human race.[18] The impact of a SNP will be determined by its position in the coding sequence.

The basic unit of DNA coding is a triplet of bases known as a codon. Each codon represents a specific amino acid. The maximum number of codons using four different bases is 64, which is considerably greater than the 20 amino acids required for protein synthesis. There is therefore a degree of duplication or redundancy, that is the code is said to be 'degenerate'. When there are multiple codons coding for one amino acid they are referred to as synonymous codons. There are also punctuation codes; that is, stop and start codons. Sometimes a mutation in base pairing occurs in a section of genome, which results in the incorrect insertion (I), or deletion (D) of one or more nucleotides. Patients may be homozygous (II or DD) or heterozygous (ID) for either of these polymorphisms. There are a number of possible outcomes if one or more base substitutions occur. If by chance, a base substitution results in the production of a synonymous exon then there is no change in amino acid sequence and no change in phenotype (the phenotype is the expression or result of a particular genotype). Alternatively, a mis-sense mutation occurs whereby a different amino acid may be inserted which results in transcription of a protein with abnormal function. In the case of an enzyme this may be reflected in decreased activity. On the other hand, the amino acid may not be in or near a functional domain of the protein, which again may not significantly impair function. More serious non-sense mutations resulting in a so-called 'null allele' are caused by the encryption of a punctuation codon, or, if the number of bases inserted is other than a multiple of three, then the entire exonic sequence downstream of the mutation is seriously disrupted resulting in a catastrophically flawed, that is, non-functional protein. This particular mutation is referred to as a 'frameshift'.[19] The recent extensive mapping of SNPs, sometimes referred to as the 'snip revolution', promises to unlock much valuable information regarding disease aetiology and will provide researchers with a vast array of targets for new treatments.[20]

Interindividual Variability in Drug Response

The understanding of pharmacogenomics may be approached by considering the effect of genetic variation on pharmacokinetics and pharmacodynamics.

Pharmacokinetic variability

The term 'pharmacokinetic variability' refers to variability in the amount of drug delivered to a receptor, otherwise known as drug disposition. Drug concentration depends on a number of factors including absorption, distribution, metabolism and elimination. Conventional pharmacogenetics has tended to concentrate on interindividual or interracial differences in drug metabolism. Historically, this has involved primarily hereditary perturbations of metabolism, caused by abnormal enzymes resulting in toxicity due to high blood levels. Latterly however, there have been exciting insights into genetic variation in processes controlling drug absorption and distribution. Furthermore, drug receptors have received attention following a realization that these could also be affected by genetic factors (i.e. SNPs) altering drug efficacy. Any individual may have a number of permutations of these factors, which may result in numerous phenotypes. An illustrative example of such a situation is given in Figure 1.1. The ever-increasing number of recognized SNPs has led to the realization that each individual may handle any medication differently and that only by *a priori* genetic testing can treatment be optimized, in other words, personalized therapy.

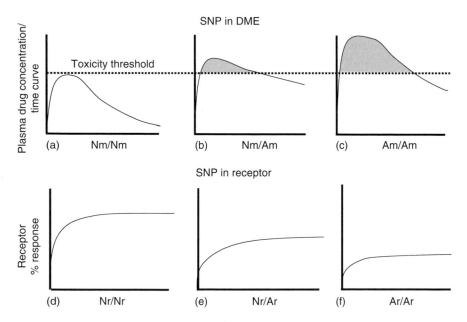

Figure 1.1 Drug disposition and effect may be influenced in a number of ways by gene abnormalities. In (a) the plasma drug concentration in a patient homozygous for the normal variant of drug metabolizing enzyme (DME) is shown. The plasma concentration never reaches the threshold for toxicity. In (b) drug disposition is depicted for a patient heterozygous for an abnormal variant. In (c) an individual homozygous for the abnormal allele, the inability of the patient to metabolize leads to toxicity. Such patients are designated poor metabolizers (PMs). In the case of a pro-drug such as codeine, the active component is not formed and the patient is a non-responder. SNPs in receptors such as the μ opioid receptor on the other hand, lead to decreased response of the receptor irrespective of plasma drug concentration. Response curve (d) shows a normal response while (e) depicts that of a heterozygote and (f) that of a homozygote for the abnormal gene. Any permutation of these SNPs may lead to a number of responses varying between normal response/no toxicity on one hand to little response/severe toxicity on the other. Nm: Normal metabolism; Am: Abnormal metabolism; Nr: Normal response; Ar: Abnormal response.

Drug metabolizing enzymes

Metabolism converts foreign substances or 'xenobiotics', which include drugs and the majority of anaesthetic agents, into water-soluble metabolites, by the introduction of small polar groups on to the parent drug. These are then more readily excreted. The responsible enzymes, commonly referred to as xenobiotic metabolizing enzymes (XMEs) or drug metabolizing enzymes (DMEs), may convert an inactive substance (e.g. codeine) into one which is pharmacologically active (in this case morphine). They may however, produce a toxic or even carcinogenic metabolite. Variation in the activity of these metabolizing enzymes may therefore carry a biological advantage or disadvantage depending on the substance being metabolized. In the case of a poorly metabolized drug that is in itself active, poor metabolism will lead to accumulation and potential toxicity. In the case of a substance that is a pro-drug like codeine, an attenuated drug effect would be expected (Fig. 1.1). Traditional pharmacology has classified pathways of metabolism as being either phase-I or phase-II reactions. Phase-I reactions consist primarily of oxidation, reduction and hydrolysis.[21] Typically but not necessarily, a phase-I reaction will precede a phase-II reaction. In the case of morphine metabolism for example, glucuronidation is not preceded by a phase-I reaction.

Phase-I P450 enzymes. The CYP P450 enzymes, a superfamily of microsomal DMEs, are the most important of the enzymes that catalyse phase-I metabolism. The advances in molecular biology which have taken place over recent decades have allowed the characterization and classification of these enzymes based upon their amino acid structure. Enzymes with more than 40% amino acid homology are grouped together in a single superfamily (the term superfamily denotes the fact that there is no species boundary). This is designated by a number, for example CYP2. If amino acid homology is greater than 55% the enzymes are grouped together in a subfamily, designated by a capital letter, for example CYP2E.[22] In the 18 superfamilies which exist in humans, enzymes belonging to superfamilies 1–4 are those which are involved in the breakdown of drugs, pollutants and chemicals. Of these superfamilies, 1–3 are the most important. It has been estimated that 90% of drug and xenobiotic metabolism can be attributed to six main enzymes CYP 1A2, 2C9, 2C19, 2D6, 2E1 and 3A4.[23] CYP enzymes are found primarily in the liver but have also been identified in the lungs, kidneys, gut and brain.[23,24]

The role of this multienzyme system, which has evolved over millennia in plants and animals, is an evolutionary consequence of plant–animal warfare. Plants synthesized chemicals for self-protection, and animals had to develop XMEs such as CYP P450 for the detoxication of these chemicals.[25]

It can now be considered as an adaptive response to environmental challenges, in that exposure to a toxic or noxious substance results in the expression of enzymes responsible for the metabolism of the particular toxin. For the most part this is a beneficial response, but it may also result in the formation of a substance that is either harmful or even carcinogenic.[26] P450 enzymes are interesting in two important respects. First of all they are inducible and secondly there are various genotypes that encrypt various forms (i.e. polymorphisms), each of which has its own particular activity. The common variant of the enzyme (sometimes referred to as wild type) is designated by the convention *1. Abnormal variants, that is enzymes whose genes have various alleles, have a corresponding number attached (e.g. CYP2A6*2). Occasionally an abnormal enzyme is produced not by an error in DNA coding but by the process of gene splicing (this is an alternative or differential form of transcription), the process by which the genetic code is transcribed to messenger RNA (mRNA). Recent work has shown that a number of different mRNAs may be transcribed from a single parent gene (i.e. one gene may code for several proteins).[27]

All of the P450 enzymes involved in drug metabolism, with the exception of CYP3A4, have a number of SNPs which have been described and characterized. The most important of these however belong to the CYP2 family of enzymes.

Pharmacogenomics of Phase-I Metabolism

CYP2D6 (codeine, tramadol)

In some respects, CYP2D6 is the prototypical P450 enzyme as far as pharmacogenomics is concerned. It was the first to be studied in detail and represents one of the best understood examples of interindividual variation among the CYP enzymes. The variation in enzyme activity first came to light when researchers studying the hypotensive drug debrisoquine noted that some subjects had an exaggerated response to treatment. Subjects with the abnormal phenotype had higher urinary concentrations of the drug and lower concentrations of its metabolite, in other words a high metabolic ratio. Subsequently, a similar situation was recorded with a second drug sparteine, a drug used both as an antidysrhythmic and oxytocic.[28] Similarly abnormal metabolic ratios were recorded. In 1982 Eichelbaum noted that the metabolic ratios of the two drugs were identical and proposed that the enzyme responsible for the metabolism of the two drugs was the same.[29] Originally designated as debrisoquine 4-hydroxylase, it was renamed CYP2D6 following sequence analysis and classification.[30] It is now recognized that between 6% and 10% of

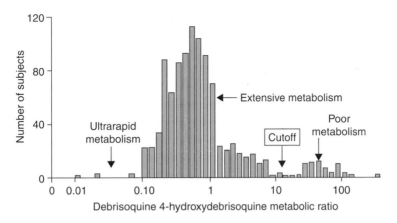

Figure 1.2 Urinary metabolic ratios of debrisoquine to its metabolite, 4-hydroxydebrisoquine, are shown for 1011 Swedish subjects. The cutoff box indicates the cutoff point between subjects with poor metabolism as a result of decreased or absent CYP2D6 activity and subjects with extensive metabolism. Modified from Yue Q et al.[32] with the permission of the publisher.

Caucasian subjects have a mutation or polymorphism at the CYP2D6 locus, which results in the production of a 'poor metabolizer' (PM) as opposed to an 'extensive metabolizer' (EM) phenotype. CYP2D6 is one of the most important XMEs and is responsible for the breakdown of a number of commonly used substances including the β-blocker metoprolol, the antidepressive nortriptyline and a number of opiates including codeine and dextromethorphan.[23,31] Interestingly, in contrast to the PM phenotype, there is a genetic variation, occuring in some Caucasian, Middle Eastern and African populations, which has been shown to produce an 'ultrarapid metabolizing' phenotype (URM). This phenotype results in abnormally high levels of morphine being produced from codeine. Such patients rapidly present with morphine-associated side effects when given standard doses of codeine.[32] The abnormality is due to gene duplication (Fig. 1.2).

Improvements in cellular biological techniques have permitted the construction of artificial or complementary DNA (cDNA) as well as the ability to clone the gene that expresses the enzyme. Over the preceding decade these advances have enabled researchers to characterize at least 70 variants of the enzyme, which are responsible for reduced activity (Table 1.2).[33]

CYP2C9 and warfarin

Warfarin is a commonly used anticoagulant. It has the disadvantage of having a rather narrow therapeutic index, which necessitates regular monitoring of its effect using, most commonly, the International Normalized

Table 1.2 Some genes, and their respective alleles, which may alter drug disposition. (A comprehensive list may be found at http://www.imm.ki.se/CYPalleles) The mutation describes the respective base substitution and the number denotes the position of the base relative to the first base of the initiation coding sequence. A mutation upstream, that is, in the promoter sequence is designated by (−). The convention C > G signifies that C is replaced by G. (Antonarakis SE. Recommendations for a nomenclature system for human gene mutations. Nomenclature Working Group. Hum Mutat 1998; 11: 1–3.) The increased activity of CYP2D6*2 is caused by gene duplication ($N = 1$–13)

Enzyme	Allele	Allele frequency	Mutation	Effect	Substrate	Reference
P450 Enzymes						
CYP1A2	CYP1A2*1C	23% Japanese	−3858 G > A	Decreased	Propanolol, Caffeine, Ondansetron, Haloperidol	23
	CYP1A2*1F		−164 C > A	Higher inducibility		
CYP2A6	CYP2A6*2	15% Chinese	479 T > A	Inactive	Nicotine, Coumarin	42–44
	CYP2A6*4A		Gene deletion	Inactive		
	CYP2A6*5		1436 G > T	Inactive		
CYP2C9	CYP2C9*2	1–3% Caucasians PMs	430 C > T	Decreased	Warfarin, NSAIDS, Diclofenac, Glipizide Tolbutamide	34–36
	CYP2C9*3		1075 A > C	Decreased		
	CYP2C9*5		1080 C > G	Decreased		
CYP2C19	CYP2C19*2	15–20% Asians PMs	Splicing defect	Inactive	Phenytoin, Mephentoin Proguanil, Proton-pump inhibitors,	38–40
	CYP2C19*3	3–5% Caucasians PMs	636 G > A	Inactive		
	CYP2C19*4		1 A > G	Inactive		
	CYP2C19*5		1297 C > T	Inactive		
	CYP2C19*6		395 G > A	Inactive		
	CYP2C19*7		Splicing defect	Inactive		
	CYP2C19*8		358 T > C	Inactive		
CYP2D6	CYP2D6*2XN	5–10% Caucasians PMs	1661 G > C	Increased activity	Codeine, Antipsychotics Propafenone, Antidysrhythmics, Metoprolol Tramadol, Antidepressants	23, 31–33
	CYP2D6*12	<29% East Africans	124 G > A	Inactive		
	CYP2D6*13		Hybrid spliceome	Inactive		
	CYP2D6*14		1785 G > A	Inactive		
	CYP2D6*15		138 insertion T	Inactive		
	CYP2D6*16		Hybrid spliceome	Inactive		
	CYP2D6*17		1023 C > T	Inactive		

Enzyme	Allele	Frequency	Variant	Effect	Substrate drugs	Reference
CYP2E1	CYP2E1*1D CYP2E1*2	Rare	8 Repeats in the 5 flanking region 1132 G > A	Increased activity Reduced activity	Fluorinated hydrocarbons, Alcohol	49–51
Phase-II enzymes						
TPMT (thiopurine methyl transferase)	TPMT*2 TPMT*3A TPMT*3C	1:300 patients are homozygous. 10% have intermediate activity	238 G > C 460 G > A 719 G > A	Severe haematopoietic toxicity	Azathioprine, 6-mercaptopurine	58–60
NAT-1 (N-acetyl transferase)	Multiple	52% white Americans	Multiple		Isoniazid, Procainamide, Hydralazine	63–65
NAT-2	Multiple		Multiple			
UGT (UDP-glucuronosyl transferase)					Irinotecan, Zidovudine, Valproic acid	53–56
UGT 1A1	UGT1A1*28	11% among whites 1% Japanese	TA × 7 repeat	Reduced metabolism Severe toxicity (irinotecan)	Bilirubin (Gilbert's syndrome)	
UGT 2B7	Various		Various	See text	Morphine	57

Ratio (INR) with concomitant alteration of drug dosage. Excessive blood concentrations of the drug may cause serious haemorrhage and therefore, must be avoided. Clinically, it is difficult to predict *a priori* what the correct starting dose should be for each patient. This is due to large interindividual differences in warfarin metabolism. Warfarin consists of a racemic mixture of both (R) and (S) enantiomers, of which the latter is more important. (S)-warfarin is metabolized to 7-hydroxywarfarin by CYP2C9.[34] A number of variants of the enzyme including CYP2C9*2 and *3 are associated with both a reduced capacity to metabolize warfarin[35] together with a lower maintenance dose.[36] Other drugs metabolized by CYP2C9 include non-steroidal anti-inflammatory drugs (NSAIDs), COX-2 selective inhibitors, the hypoglycaemic agent tolbutamide, phenytoin and the angiotensin-II receptor antagonist losartan.[37]

CYP2C19 (proton-pump inhibitors)

The hepatic enzyme CYP2C19 has also a number of SNPs which have interracial differences in expression pattern. Of these, CYP2C19*2 and CYP2C19*3 are best characterized. CYP2C19*2 occurs in 25% of the Asian population in comparison to 13% of Caucasians, while the CYP2C19*3 allele occurs in 8% of Asians in comparison with 1% of Caucasians. Those patients who are homozygous for the inactive or 'null' alleles of CYP2C19 are highly sensitive to substrates of the enzyme such as diazepam, the proton-pump inhibitor omeprazole, propanolol and the antidepressive amitriptyline.[38] An important clinical example of abnormal metabolism of one of its substrates involves the proton-pump inhibitor omeprazole. In one study, which compared the association between genotype and efficacy of eradication of *Helicobacter pylori*, it was shown that those with an EM genotype fared less well in terms of eradication of the organism in comparison to those subjects who were heterozygous for the PM gene.[39] This is an unusual example of a pharmacological advantage resulting from a mutation of a gene controlling a CYP enzyme. Another interesting example involves the antimalarial drug proguanil, which is converted to its active metabolite by CYP2C19. A study carried out among the inhabitants of the island of Vanuatu in Polynesia discovered that 70% of the population were PMs for the drug, a fact which could have serious consequences for malaria prophylaxis in the region.[40]

CYP2A6 and the pharmacogenomics of smoking

There has been considerable interest in the metabolism of nicotine and the role of differential nicotine metabolism in initiation and maintenance of nicotine addiction. In 1997 it was reported that the hepatic enzyme CYP2A6 (previously known as coumarin 7-hydroxylase) was the major catalyst of nicotine inactivation to cotinine by C-oxidation.[41] Subsequently it was discovered that there were functional variants of this enzyme, which were possibly related to different levels of addiction between individuals.[42] In addition, it was recognized that there was a lower incidence of two null alleles of CYP2A6, namely CYP2A6*2 and CYP2A6*3 in a tobacco dependent population. Nicotine addicts adjust their smoking to maintain constant nicotine levels and therefore, individuals with impaired metabolism need to smoke fewer cigarettes, and even smokers who are heterozygous for the CYP2A6 null-allele need significantly fewer cigarettes. Ethnic differences in nicotine metabolism have also been found which are related to different activities of CYP2A6. Chinese–Americans absorbed less nicotine per cigarette and metabolized nicotine more slowly than whites or Latinos and have a lower incidence of lung cancers.[43] A number of different alleles of CYP2A6 have now been identified and attempts have been made to correlate the incidence of these genetic variants with both smoking and lung cancer rates.[44] In an attempt to mimic the genetic advantage of the null allele by using enzyme blockers to impair CYP2A6 nicotine breakdown, researchers have successfully altered smoking behaviour. It was found that smokers whose nicotine metabolism was impaired using the enzyme blockers tranylcypromine and methoxalen, required fewer cigarettes and had a longer latent period between cigarettes.[45] It is possible that other CYP enzymes are also involved in the psychopharmacology of smoking. CYP2D6 for example, has been suggested to modify smoking behaviour through an effect on the metabolism of central transmitters such as dopamine.[46]

CYP2E1 and volatile anaesthetic agents

The CYP2E1 isoenzyme is induced both by smoking[47] and by the intake of alcohol.[48] There are a number of polymorphisms which have been described.[49] Virtually all volatile anaesthetic agents are metabolized by this enzyme.[50,51] It has been suggested that variations in the activity of this enzyme may explain some of the differences in outcome from anaesthesia and in particular the occurrence of postoperative nausea and vomiting (PONV).[52] It may also explain the individual propensity to develop anaesthetic related complications, such as jaundice, which are known to be associated with the metabolism of volatile agents.

Pharmacogenomics of Phase-II Metabolism

Phase-II metabolism completes the solubilization process which may involve one or other of a number of chemical steps. These include methylation, glucuronidation, sulphation and acetylation.

Glucuronidation

Glucuronidation is catalysed by the enzyme uridine diphosphate-glucuronosyl transferase (UGT). UGTs are glycoproteins, localized in the endoplasmic reticulum and nuclear membrane. Around 24 human UGT genes have been identified. Individual variation has been found in five of these isoforms.[53] One important member of this group of enzymes is the UGT2B7 isoform, which is involved in the glucuronidation of a number of physiologically important substances including steroid hormones, bile acids, retinoids and fatty acids as well as a number of commonly used drugs such as the anticonvulsant valproic acid, NSAIDS and the antiviral agent zidovudine.[54,55] It is also of particular importance to the anaesthetist because of its central role in the breakdown of morphine and codeine.[56] A number of polymorphisms of this enzyme have been described. In one study, cancer patients receiving morphine were genotyped at the UGT2B7 locus and simultaneous measurement made of metabolic ratios of morphine versus morphine–3- and morphine–6-glucuronide (M3G, M6G). Of the 12 polymorphisms found at UGT2B7 locus, only one was found in the protein coding sequence. Although there was considerable variation in metabolic ratios, it was felt that because there was a unimodal distribution of these ratios (i.e. unlike the typical bi- or trimodal distribution seen with P450 enzymes such as CYP2D6), factors other than polymorphisms were exerting an influence (Table 1.2).[57]

Thiopurine S-methyl transferase (TPMT)

The genetic variation in TPMT activity is an important example of how pharmacogenomics may influence the outcome of treatment. TPMT is an important enzyme involved in the metabolism of a number of chemotherapeutic agents used in the treatment of acute lymphatic leukaemia and a number of autoimmune conditions such as rheumatoid arthritis and myasthenia gravis as well as in the prevention of rejection following organ transplantation.[58] Thiopurine substrates of TPMT include 6-mercaptopurine, thioguanine and azathioprine. Several studies have shown that patients with low enzyme activity are at high risk of serious, if not potentially fatal haematopoetic toxicity if treated with conventional doses of these drugs.[59] TPMT exhibits polymorphism with around 10% of the population at intermediate risk due to heterozygosity and 1 in 300 at high risk due to homozygosity of the abnormal gene.[60] The commonest alleles for TPMT are TPMT*2 and TPMT*3 which are more labile than the wild-type enzyme.[61] Genotyping for the abnormal allele of TPMT has become a standard procedure in some centres prior to commencement of therapy. When TPMT deficiency is diagnosed thiopurine medication is reduced by on average

90%.[62] In this way, optimal therapy in all patients with acute lymphatic leukaemia is guaranteed.

N-acetyl transferase (NAT)

A large number of commonly used drugs are metabolized by NAT including some antibiotics. The acetylation polymorphism, that is the slow-acetylator status, to which reference, with respect to isoniazid, has already been made, is among the most common of DME mutations. More than 50% of individuals in Caucasian populations are homozygous for a recessive trait and are therefore designated 'slow-acetylators' (i.e. PMs). They are less efficient than 'rapid-acetylators' in the metabolism of numerous drugs including isoniazid, environmental and industrial chemicals. In addition to isoniazid-induced neuropathy, patients with the abnormality may also present with procainamide-induced lupus, sulphonamide-induced hypersensitivity, and dye-associated bladder cancer.[63,64] There are two NAT genes in humans which have been designated NAT1 and NAT2.[65] Apart from associations with cancer there is also a link between the polymorphism and chemical-induced asthma.[66]

Carrier Proteins (Membrane Transporters)

Membrane transport proteins play a fundamental role in a number of physiological processes. Until recently it was assumed that drug transport across membranes was primarily determined by molecular weight and lipophilicity. Recently it has been recognized that a group of proteins called transporters that span the lipid bilayer of the cell membrane play a crucial role in drug transport.[67] Transporters may be either passive, such as ion channels and the glucose transporter, or active, which requires energy. One important class of ATP-powered transport proteins is larger and more diverse than the other classes and is referred to as the ATP-binding cassette (ABC), a superfamily of more than 100 proteins that are found in organisms ranging from bacteria to humans. One of these transporters is called the P-glycoprotein multidrug transporter (PGP).[68] It should be noted that some of these proteins and the respective genes have dual nomenclature. For example, P-PGP is expressed by the multidrug resistant gene (MDR1), which is synonymous with ABC B1 (an attempt has been made by the ABC Subcommittee of the Human Genome Gene Nomenclature Committee to bring order and consistency to the subject). Details of this nomenclature can be found at www.gene.ucl.ac.uk/ nomenclature/genefamily/abc.html.

Table 1.3 Some drugs which are substrates of P-glycoprotein. The uptake and distribution of these drugs including transport across the blood–brain barrier will be affected by mutations in the MDR/PGP gene

Anticancer drugs	HIV protease inhibitors	Calcium-channel blockers
Doxorubicin	Indinavir	Diltiazem
Topotecan	Nelfinavir	Verapamil
Vinblatine	Saquinavir	
Vincristine		
		H1 antagonists
Cardiac drugs	**Antibiotics**	Fexofenadine
Digoxin	Erythromycin	Terfenadine
Quinidine		
		H2 antagonists
Anti-emetics	**β-blockers**	Cimetidine
Domperidone	Celiprolol	Ranitidine
Ondansetron	Talinolol	
		Analgesics
		Morphine

The PGP transporter was initially studied in the context of cancer chemotherapy. It has been recognized for some time that this transporter is responsible for the removal of chemotherapeutic agents from cells and the development of the phenomenon of multidrug resistance in tumour cells. This transporter is found in a number of locations in the body such as liver, gut and kidney and is also present at the blood–brain barrier. Several mutations have been found in the gene that codes for this protein, one of which (at position 3435 in the gene) is associated with altered blood concentrations of a number of drugs including digoxin, anti-cancer drugs, HIV protease inhibitors, β-blockers and antihistamines (Table 1.3).[69,70]

Recently drug movement across the blood–brain barrier has been found to be largely dependent on drug transporters. There are huge therapeutic implications for the future of drug development in this area given that it is possible to both induce and inhibit PGP by a number of medications currently available and thereby modulate the function of drugs acting on the central nervous system (CNS). Fexofenadine is a metabolite of the commonly used antihistamine terfenadine and has been found to be a high affinity probe for PGP and can be used to assess the transporter activity in patients. Using this probe, researchers found that it was possible to correlate drug plasma concentrations with MDR genotype.[71] An important pharmacogenomic example of this is in the context of HIV therapy, where it has been shown that PGP polymorphisms correlate with plasma protease-inhibitor concentrations in patients undergoing treatment for HIV.[72] By using pharmacological blockers of PGP it may be possible to enhance therapy of HIV infection.[73] Recent research has revealed a key role for the

Table 1.4 Some diseases associated with SNPs of transporter genes

Condition	Transporter	Name	Reference
Alzheimer's disease	5-HTT	Serotonin transporter	74
Breast cancer	THTR 1, 2	Thiamine transporter	79
Cystic fibrosis	CFTR	Cystic fibrosis transmembrane conductance regulator	75
Gastro-intestinal disease (inflammatory and malignant)	PGP	P-glycoprotein	77
Immune response	PGP	(P-glycoprotein)	80
Parkinson's disease	DAT	Dopamine transporter	78
Stress/depression	5-HTT	Serotonin transporter	76

wider family of transporters in a number of diverse conditions such as Alzheimer's disease,[74] cystic fibrosis,[75] stress/depression,[76] gastro-intestinal disease,[77] and Parkinson's disease.[78] There have also been recent associations with breast cancer[79] and the immune system (Table 1.4).[80]

Cystic fibrosis is a condition caused by a defect in the membrane transporter ABCC7, originally designated the cystic fibrosis transmembrane conductance regulator (CFTR) gene. This transporter also plays a role in the aetiology of various types of diarrhoea including those of infective origin. Both the gene and its product have therefore become attractive targets for modulation by drugs. Recently the product of the CFTR gene has been studied in animals. Gene-knockout mice, that is mice without the CFTR gene, bred to mimic cystic fibrosis, are unable to contract cholera. It was proposed that a chemical designed to block CFTR would mimic these gene-knockout mice. Thiazolidinone is such a compound and is non-toxic to humans and mice. When given to mice infected with cholera the intestinal secretions were reduced by 90%.[81] Given that on average a million people die each year from the dehydrating effects of infective diarrhoea the potential impact of such novel therapies is immense.

At present there is ongoing research into the possibility of beneficially altering the product of the CFTR gene in cystic fibrosis sufferers. This may be possible by using the latest recombinant DNA technologies.[82]

Unlike cystic fibrosis, which has an unequivocal genetic basis, many common diseases such as depression, hypertension and diabetes are the result of the interaction of a number of genes with an environmental trigger. Depression is a common condition, which typifies gene–environmental interaction. A number of neurotransmitters such as serotonin, norepineph-rine and dopamine, as well as the opioid receptor, sex hormones, the gamma amino butyric acid (GABA) pathway and brain P450 enzymes (CYP2D6) have been incriminated in its aetiology and are all logical targets for pharmacotherapy. In particular, the serotonin transporter has proved to be a fruitful area for study as has its controlling gene (5-HTT gene). The activity of the transporter determines the synaptic concentration of sero-tonin. The 5-HTT gene displays polymorphism in its regulatory region (i.e. the promoter region), which consists of a 44-base-pair insertion. The presence or absence of this insertion has been shown to be a predictive marker of response to treatment with reuptake inhibitors (SSRIs, selective serotonin reuptake inhibitors) such as fluvoxamine and paroxetine.[76]

Pharmacodynamic Variability

Pharmacodynamics refers to the relationship between concentration and its effect. Individuals with identical plasma concentrations of a given drug may vary in their response, indicating that mechanisms other than phar-macokinetics are involved. Recent breakthroughs in molecular biological research have facilitated the description of mutations in genes coding for a number of important biological receptors. The standard methodology for interpreting drug action is the dose–response curve. The effect of a mutation in the receptor protein is effectively to alter the affinity for either a receptor agonist or antagonist. The effects of a reduction in affinity for an agonist are schematically outlined in Figure 1.1.

Receptors

Genetic polymorphisms have been found to be associated with a number of key areas related to anaesthesia including pain thresholds and the resulting requirements for analgesia. A much quoted polymorphism is that described by Bond and co-workers which consists of a SNP at pos-ition 118 of the μ opioid receptor gene in 10% of the population in their study.[83] The variant protein was three times more potent in its interaction with β-endorphin than with the wild-type allele. This may have implica-tions for determining both the need for, and the response to opioid anal-gesics. In addition, SNPs of the μ opioid receptor may help to identify individuals predisposed to opiate addiction. Similarly SNPs have been described for a number of other important drug targets such as the recep-tor for oestrogen,[84] dopamine[85] and 5-hydroxytryptamine (5HT-1, -2).[86] The ryanodine receptor (RYR1) is an essential component of the calcium homeostasis of skeletal muscle in mammals. In humans, mutations in the

RYR1 gene have been associated with various muscle disorders including malignant hyperthermia and central core disease.[87]

Blood pressure regulation is determined by the interplay of a number of well-characterized interdependent control systems. Within each of these systems, multiple genes are expressed, each of which will contribute to the separate control system and which are synchronized with each other to regulate blood pressure. At present it is unknown how and to what extent the different genes contribute to this system, how they interact with one another and how they are influenced by environmental factors and by lifestyle. However, modern tools, which enable the investigation or simultaneous study of a large number of genes, together with linkage studies using a high number of SNP markers promise to reveal the gene variations that cause inherited hypertension. Until now there have been few reports of any single gene being associated with an alteration in treatment outcome. However, there is a DD variant of the angiotensin converting enzyme, (ACE) which has been found to be associated with response to treatment with ACE inhibitors[88] as well as being a positive predictor for left ventricular hypertrophy.[89]

Another example of varied drug response due to mutations in receptors concerns asthma, which is a complex syndrome, typifying environmental–gene interactions and characterized by a varied and unpredictable response to treatment. Although, at present, there are no data to indicate that asthma itself can be attributed to β-2-adrenergic (β-2-AR) polymorphisms, there are convincing data to suggest that specific variants of this gene are associated with adrenergic receptor down-regulation,[90] greater asthma severity,[91] and enhanced reversibility.[92] Recently, it has been shown that polymorphisms exist both at receptor level and at the level of the promoter region of the 5-lipoxygenase gene (ALOX5 gene), which controls leukotriene synthesis.[93] Subjects homozygous, or heterozygous for the wild-type allele, had a greater improvement in forced expiratory volume in 1 second (FEV1), when treated with an oral 5-lipoxygenase inhibitor, than did subjects who possessed the variant alleles.[94]

Other common conditions where a genetic marker has been used to indicate a possible modification in therapy include diabetes,[95] schizophrenia[96] and Alzheimer's disease.[97] These conditions typify polygenic illness where a gene may indicate a given propensity to develop the illness but is not pathognomonic of that illness. Finally, an interesting but rare mutation in an ion channel concerns the potassium voltage-gated channel, which is associated with the long QT syndrome and may be a cause of a fatal dysrhythmia, namely *Torsade-de-pointes* especially in the presence of certain drugs such as antihistamines or anti-emetics such as droperidol (Table 1.5).[98]

Table 1.5 A selection of gene SNPs which may result in altered transmitter/receptor status

Receptor	Name	Reference	Drug	Associated condition	Drug effect associated with SNP
APOE4	Apolipoprotein E	97	Tacrine	Alzheimer's disease	Variation in cognitive function improvement
OPRM1	μ opioid receptor	83	Opioid analgesics	Analgesia, opioid addiction	Altered pain threshold. Increased addiction propensity
5-HT1, 5HT2	Hydroxytryptamine receptor	86	Antipsychotics (e.g. fluvoxamine)	Schizophrenia	Response to treatment
D1, D2, D3, D4	Dopamine receptor	85	Antipsychotics	Schizophrenia	Altered response to treatment, incidence of side effects
β-2AR	β-2 adrenergic receptor	91–92	β-2 agonists	Asthma	Susceptibility to receptor down-regulation
HERG/MIRP/KCNH2	Potassium voltage-gated channel	98	Terfenadine, droperidol	Long QT syndrome	Torsade-de-pointes
SUR1	Sulphonylurea receptor	95	Hypoglycaemic agents	Diabetes mellitus	Sulphonylurea-induced insulin release
ER alpha	Oestrogen receptor alpha	84	Oestrogen therapy	Osteoporosis	Increase in bone mineral
LTC4	Leukotriene receptor	93	Leukotriene receptor antagonists, for example montelukast	Asthma	Altered treatment response
ALOX5	5-Lipoxygenase	94	Leukotriene-receptor antagonists	Asthma	Improved FEV1
RYR1	Ryanodine receptor	87	Volatile anaesthetic agents	Malignant hyperthermia	Increased risk of malignant hyperthermia
ACE	Angiotensin converting enzyme	88–89	ACE inhibitors (e.g. enalapril)	Hypertension/ventricular hypertrophy	Renoprotective effect, blood pressure reduction, reduced left ventricular mass

Pharmacogenomics and Drug Development

Background

The primary goal of pharmaceutical companies in the genomic era is to convert genome-based knowledge into new medications. The first step in drug development is to find key targets (established or novel); that is, genes that code for proteins that are involved in disease processes. The next step is to find and test substances that can beneficially modify or modulate the target. Gene identification is a complicated process, which includes the evaluation and comparison of DNA sequences from a number of other organisms whose genomes have already been partially or completely sequenced. Much of this information exists in small, distinct sequences based upon lengths of artificial DNA called 'expressed sequence tags' (ESTs). This complementary or cDNA is created directly from mRNA using the enzyme reverse transcriptase and is therefore devoid of intronic or non-coding sequences. The key technological discovery which has facilitated genome sequencing is the polymerase chain reaction (PCR) which facilitates the amplification of minute amounts of DNA, which in turn can be isolated and sequenced.

Bioinformatics

Functional genomics is the science of attributing a function to a genomic sequence. This can be done by mining existing EST databases for sequences already catalogued and characterized. This novel type of gene-hunting known as 'in silico research' is called bioinformatics. Bioinformatics utilizes a number of sophisticated computer algorithms, as well as standard mathematical and statistical tools to allow putative interspecies comparisons of genes, which may have a common evolutionary source and may have both a conserved relative position on the genome and a common function. Conserved gene order between species is called 'synteny' and those genes with similar function are called 'orthologues'. The key in this type of analysis is to detect or predict relationships with sufficient confidence that structural or functional information about a known sequence can be sensibly and justifiably transferred to an unknown one. This use of interspecies comparison of genes is called 'phylogenomics',[99] a discipline that has become an indispensable part of new drug discovery.[100] In addition, there are also databases containing thousands of protein–amino acid sequences which hold the key to the elucidation of disease processes and which may act as targets for new therapies. This is the basis for proteomics-based research.[101]

Databases, which are held in a number of institutions, both public and private, and now in the public domain, are readily accessible to researchers who may wish to deposit new sequence data, or for the purpose of genomic-based research. These databases are continually being updated and expanded. There are three main data banks for DNA sequences. These are GenBank database at the National Centre for Biotechnology Information (NCBI) in the US, the DNA databank of Japan (DDBJ) and European Bioinformatics Institute (EBI) at the European Molecular Biology Laboratory (EMBL). These organizations liase with each other on a daily basis, resulting in a databank of comprehensive information which is readily available to researchers. This plethora of data, which is estimated to double in size every 9–12 months, is categorized both by species and by data type.

Microarrays and studies of gene expression

The second major technological advance in drug development has been the recently acquired ability to study patterns of gene expression in disease and following exposure to a drug or toxin. In other words, gene expression analysis can be used both to define gene targets and to investigate new agents. For example, in a condition such as sepsis or cancer there is a consistent and characteristic pattern of gene expression, which may be regarded as typical of that condition that is, its signature or profile. This consists of differential gene up-regulation or down-regulation with corresponding changes in cellular protein levels. Each cell in the body is capable of producing around 15,000–25,000 proteins.[102] Typically, in an average transcriptome around 1000 proteins are identifiable. This expression pattern will be influenced in a stereotypical fashion by extraneous stimuli. This profile can then be used, for example, in the case of cancer, to analyse the key expression differences underlying malignancy. Similarly, changes in gene expression may anticipate any perceived clinical effect of drugs and for this reason the technique is used extensively by drug companies, both as a means of investigating potentially useful drugs, and as a way of understanding the mechanisms of adverse drug effects (toxicogenomics) (Table 1.6).[103]

Gene expression analysis is performed using DNA microarrays also known as gene-chips. These exist in two forms: either oligodeoxynucleotide arrays or cDNA chips. An array consists of thousands of microscopic single stranded spots of this cDNA, amplified by PCR and immobilized on a solid support such as glass or silicon. This is called a probe. When creating a microarray, a spectrum of genes can be selected which are appropriate to the study being performed (e.g. inflammation, cancer and drug response). The microarray may take the form of many

Table 1.6 Definitions of some terms used in drug development

Genomics	The study of the genome. This includes gene structure and function as well as control mechanisms, the transcriptome, gene expression, gene–environment interactions and the wider implications of gene contribution to disease
Functional genomics	The study of the role of genes and their products in health and disease. At present it is extensively used by pharmaceutical companies in their quest for novel medications
Reverse genomics	An alternative to traditional or *sequence-driven* drug research. In reverse genomics the phenotype of laboratory animals is altered using gene-knockout techniques using chemicals or RNA interference (siRNA)
Pharmacogenetics	The study of the influence of single genes on drug response
Toxicogenomics	The study of adverse effects of xenobiotics, for example drugs, primarily using microarray technology to analyse gene expression
Pharmacogenomics	The study of the influence of the entire genome on drug response and the impact of genomic information on drug discovery
Bioinformatics	The use of computers to analyse DNA sequences held in databases (*in silico* 'mining' of databases) to facilitate the identification of gene function and therapeutic targets
Proteomics	The study of the function of the entire protein product of the genome.
Pharmacoproteomics	The study of protein–protein, and drug–protein interactions
Phylogenomics	The analysis of interspecies genomic differences
Pharmacophylogenomics	The use of microarrays to analyse and evaluate the differences in gene expression across species boundaries usually following exposure to a xenobiotic (i.e. a drug or chemical)

thousands of candidate gene samples, the sequences of which are derived from public databases such as Genbank. It is anticipated that in the foreseeable future, microarrays will be created which may encompass the entire human genome, thereby permitting, in one experiment, analysis of the entire spectrum of biological response to a given stimulus or perturbation. A typical gene chip is $1.5\,cm^2$ with 65,000 spots representing 6800 genes.[104] After the microarray has been prepared, the test sample, the target, is added to the array. Hybridization (i.e. annealing of cDNA strands) between the array and test will occur if there is a match between the two samples. In practice, two samples, one of which acts as a control, are used. Each of these is labelled with different fluorescent dyes. By analysing the colour and intensity of the fluorescence it is possible to determine whether the gene in question is either up- or down-regulated.

The applications of microarray technology are far reaching. However, at present considerable effort is being made to characterize the interspecies variation in gene expression which is a vital step before acquired animal data can be extrapolated to humans (pharmacophylogenomics).[100] It may be used to analyse differential gene expression in tumours[105] which has facilitated, in some areas, better classification and more accurate prognosis.[106] Microarrays are increasingly being used to examine gene expression in diverse areas such as sepsis,[107] infectious disease,[108] lung disease,[109] and cardiology.[110] Recently one biotech company, Roche Molecular Diagnostics, introduced a simple gene testing device, the 'Amplichip CYP450', which is essentially a microarray developed to determine the status of two genes; CYP2D6 and CYP2C19.[111] This device provides for the first time a simple test to determine the response to a number of drugs, including analgesics, antidepressants and antipsychotics.

Recent trends

The process of analysing base sequences, postulating a function for the sequence and researching this postulate (termed hypothesis-driven or inductive genomics) is currently consuming vast resources and has led to a plethora of new potential drug targets, outstripping the capacity of companies to effectively select, prioritize, develop and market new products.

Recently the concept of 'deductive' genomics has been postulated as an alternative to sequence-based pharmacological research.[112] This process involves inducing mutations in animals, particularly in mice, using chemicals such as ethyl nitrosourea (ENU) which targets A and T bases. The resulting phenotype can then be studied with the advantage of *a priori* knowledge of the genetic mutation. A similar concept of 'reverse genomics' has been used to validate gene targets using 'knockout' experiments in mice. This involves breeding genetically altered mice, in which a specific gene has been effectively switched off. One recent technology involves the use of small sections of RNA called *small interfering RNAs* (siRNA),[113] which can be used to effectively switch off or 'knock-down' genes. Various therapeutic hypotheses can then be tested using these knockout or knock-down mice, on pathways involving the complementary protein of the respective gene. Results, both interesting and unexpected, have been observed in a number of cases where association hypotheses have been confirmed.

Ethical and Legal Issues

The rapid progress in genome-based science has outstripped legal and ethical considerations of both its applications and wider social implications. The general public, as expected, have reacted with guarded scepticism to the implications of the endeavours of scientists to improve human well-being and to treat disease using so-called gene therapy. Individuals have expressed concern that genetic information could affect their access to health insurance and therefore health care.[114] On the other hand, insurers are worried that unscrupulous individuals may try to obtain financial reward on the basis of prior knowledge of disease probability.[115] At present in the UK a moratorium has been placed on the use of genetic tests to settle insurance premiums and in the US there has been recent legislation in this area (Genetic Information Non-discrimination Act of 2003) (www.genome.gov/PolicyEthics/). The acquisition of pharmacogenomics-based knowledge may create ethical dilemmas for drug companies who may wish to target some racial groups and thereby disadvantage others. Health care providers may also risk being labelled as discriminatory, if treatment is deemed inappropriate to those patients known for example, to be PMs.[116] Storage and utilization of genetic information represents another dilemma for those involved in research; should subjects, spouses or relatives be given details of all genomic data which comes to light during the course of a study or, perhaps only relevant health care providers? These and other legal, social and regulatory issues have recently been discussed in a document published in September 2003 by The Nuffield Council on Bioethics, which is available at www.nuffieldbioethics.org.

The Future

The biotech revolution, which contributed to the exaggerated swings of stock markets, due to the unrealistic expectations of investors, has now given way to a more circumspect and balanced view of the impact of genome-based medicine on the future of health care in western countries. Although to-date there has been a paucity of new drugs introduced as a direct result of the biotech boom, it is highly likely that further identification of genes (at present only around 50% of the 32,000 genes have been characterized) and improved techniques for examining, quantifying and interpreting gene expression and protein interactions at the cellular level will give rise to a new generation of medications which will be considered revolutionary. In developing economies new insights into the treatment and prevention of diarrhoeal illnesses will have a potentially major impact. The sequencing of the DNA of pathogens including bacteria and the malarial parasite[117] will also spawn new types of therapies.

Using recombinant DNA technology, drugs such as erythropoietin, recombinant human activated protein C (rhaPC) and human insulin have been introduced and greater understanding of certain cancers such as breast cancer have facilitated the introduction of drugs such as herceptin which targets the HER2 oncogene. The fuller understanding of the genome and its products such as enzymes and receptors has already impacted the use of some medications. In the case of some medications such as antidepressants, up to 50% of patients obtain no benefit from therapy. In the future it will be possible, using simple testing devices to screen patients for a number of genes, to predict not only which patients will respond to treatment but also those patients who will develop potentially serious side effects. Fuller understanding of gene networks and gene–environment interactions will continue to bring about a more rational approach to therapy in common diseases such as hypertension and asthma. Already P450 enzymes have been reclassified allowing better understanding of drug metabolism and interactions. Gene control mechanisms continue to prove to be infuriatingly complex but there have been valuable insights into enzyme induction, including identification of cellular receptors that interact with environmental substances,[118] which have important practical implications for patients. At present, pharmaceuticals currently target only 500 or so gene products.[119] The proteome consists of around 100,000 proteins. Even allowing for a large percentage of these not being involved in disease processes, it nevertheless suggests that there is an enormous untapped pool of worthwhile drug targets for potentially new therapies. Continued technological innovation will bring faster and cheaper methods for genetic analysis and routine screening for SNPs. Indeed, whole genome analysis will become a standard screening tool and provide, thereafter, all the information required by health care providers to optimize treatment for patients. The dream of individually tailored medicine has become a reality. However, the serious ethical dilemmas generated by these discoveries will have to be resolved before we can safely use these new technologies.

References

1. IHGSC (International Human Genome Sequencing Consortium). Initial sequencing of the human genome. Nature 2001; 409: 860–921.
2. CESC (The C. Elegans Sequencing Consortium). Genome sequence of the nematode C. elegans. A platform for investigating biology. Science 1998; 282: 2012–2018.
3. Ebersberger I, Metzler D, Schwarz C et al. Genomewide comparison of DNA sequences between humans and chimpanzees. Am J Hum Genet 2002; 70: 1490–1497.
4. Kirkness EF, Bafna V, Halpern AL et al. The dog genome: survey sequencing and comparative analysis. Science 2003; 301: 1898–1903.

5. Kalow W. Familial incidence of low pseudocholinesterase level. Lancet 1956; 2: 576.
6. Mendel JG. Versuche uber Pflanzen-Hybride. Verhandlungen der Naturforschenden Vereines in Brunn. 1886; 4.
7. Garrod AE. Inborn Errors of Metabolism. New York: Oxford University Press, 1909.
8. Snyder LH. Studies in human inheritance IX. The inheritance of taste deficiency in man. Ohio J Sci 1932; 32: 436–438.
9. Carson PE, Flanagan CL, Ickes CE, Alving AS. Enzymatic deficiency in primaquine-sensitive erythrocytes. Science 1956; 124: 484–485.
10. Hughes HB, Biehl JP, Jones AP. Metabolism of isoniazide in man as related to the occurrence of peripheral neuritis. Am Rev Tuberculosis 1954; 70: 266–273.
11. Motulsky AG. Drug reactions, enzymes and biochemical genetics. J Am Med Assoc 1957; 165: 835–837.
12. Kalow W. Pharmacogenetics, Heredity and the Response to Drugs. Philadelphia, London: WB Saunders, 1962.
13. Vogel F. Moderne Probleme der Humangenetik. Ergeb Innere Med Kinderheil 1959; 12: 52–125.
14. Mahgoub A, Idle JR, Dring LG et al. Polymorphic hydroxylation of debrisoquine in man. Lancet 1977; 1: 584–586.
15. Weinshilboum RM, Sladek SL. Mercaptopurine pharmacogenetics: monogenetic inheritance of erythrocyte thiopurine methyltransferase activity. Am J Hum Genet 1980; 32: 651–662.
16. Wedlund PJ, Aslanian WS, McAllister CB, Wilkinson GR et al. Mephentoin hydroxylation deficiency in Caucasians: frequency of a new oxidative drug metabolism. Clin Pharmacol Ther 1984; 36: 773–780.
17. SNP Group (The International SNP Map Working Group). A map of human genome sequence variation containing 1.42 million single nucleotide polymorphisms. Nature 2001; 409: 928–933.
18. Reich DE, Gabriel SB, Altshuler D. Quality and completeness of SNP databases. Nat Genet 2003; 33: 457–458.
19. Brown TA. Mutations, repair and recombination. In: Genomes, 2nd ed. Oxford: Bios Science Publications, 2002; 420–424.
20. Taylor JG, Choi EH, Foster CB et al. Using genetic variation to study human disease. Trend Mol Biol 2001; 7: 507–512.
21. Calvey TN, Williams NE. Principles and Practice of Pharmacology for Anaesthetists, 3rd ed. Blackwell Science, 1997; 36–69.
22. Slaughter RL, Edwards DJ. Recent advances: the cytochrome P450 enzymes. Ann Pharmacother 1995; 29: 619–624.
23. Tanaka E. Clinically important pharmacokinetic drug–drug interactions: role of cytochrome P450 enzymes. J Clin Pharm Ther 1998; 23: 403–416.
24. Miksys SL, Tyndale RF. Drug metabolising cytochrome P450 in the brain. J Psychiatry Neuroscience 2002; 27: 406–415.
25. Yang CS, Brady JF, Hong JY. Dietary effects on cytochromes P450, xenobiotic metabolism and toxicity. FASEB J 1992; 6: 737–744.
26. Wolf CR, Mahmood A, Henderson CJ, McLeod R, Manson MM, Neal GE, Hayes JD. Modulation of the cytochrome P450 system as a mechanism of chemoprotection. International Agency for Research on Cancer Scientific Publications 1996; 139: 165–173.
27. Brown TA. Synthesis and processing mRNA. In: Genomes, 2nd ed. Oxford: Bios Science Publications, 2002; 273–302.

28. Eichelbaum M, Spannbrucker N, Steincke B, Dengler HJ. Defective N-oxidation of sparteine in man, a new pharmacogenetic defect. Eur J Clin Pharmacol 1979; 16: 183–187.

29. Eichelbaum M, Bertilsson L, Sawe J, Zekorn C. Polymorphic oxidation of sparteine and debrisoquine: related pharmacogenetic entities. Clin Pharmacol Ther 1982; 2: 184–186.

30. Gonzalez FJ, Vilbois F, Hardwick JP et al. Human debrisoquine 4-hydroxylase (CYPIID1): cDNA and deduced amino acid sequence and assignment of the CYP2D locus of chromosome 22. Genomics 1988; 2: 174–179.

31. Pelkonen O, Maenpa J, Taavitsainen P, Rautio A, Raunio H. Inhibition and induction of human cytochrome P450 (CYP) enzymes. Xenobiotica 1998; 28: 1203–1253.

32. Yue Q, Alm C, Svensson J, Sawe J. Quantification of the O- and N-demethylated and the glucuronidated metabolites of codeine relative to the debrisoquine metabolic ratio in urine in ultrarapid, rapid, and poor debrisoquine hydroxylators. Ther Drug Monit 1997; 19: 539–542.

33. Kimura S, Umeno M, Skoda RC, Meyer UA, Gonzalez FJ. The human debrisoquine 4-hydroxylase (CYP2D) locus: sequence and identification of the polymorphic CYP2D6 gene, a related gene and a pseudogene. Am J Hum Genet 1989; 45: 889–904.

34. Retie AE, Korzekwa KR, Kunze KL et al. Hydroxylation of warfarin by human cDNA-expressed cytochrome P-450: a role for P-450 2C9 in the aetiology of (S)-warfarin-drug interactions. Chem Res Toxicol 1992; 5: 54–59.

35. Retie AE, Wienkers LC, Gonzalez FJ et al. Impaired s-warfarin metabolism catalysed by R144C allelic variant of CYP2C9. Pharmacogenetics 1994; 4: 39–42.

36. Linder MW, Looney S, Adams JE et al. Warfarin dose adjustment based on CYP2C9 genetic polymorphisms. J Thromb Thrombol 2002; 14: 227–232.

37. Gonzalez RD. Cytochrome P450 pharmacogenetics in drug development. In vitro studies and clinical consequences. Curr Drug Metab 2002; 3: 289–309.

38. Mancinelli L, Cronin M, Sadee W. Pharmacogenomics: the promise of personalised medicine. AAPS Pharm Sci 2000; 2: 30–37.

39. Sapone A, Vaira D, Trespidi S et al. The clinical role of cytochrome P450 genotypes in Helicobacter pylori management. Am J Gastroenterol 2003; 98: 1010–1015.

40. Koneko A, Koneko O, Taleo G et al. High frequencies of CYP2C19 mutations and poor metabolism of proguanil in Vanuatu. Lancet 1997; 349: 921–922.

41. Messina ES, Tyndale RF, Sellers EM. A major role for CYP2A6 in nicotine C-oxidation by human liver microsomes. J Pharm Exp Ther 1997; 282: 1608–1614.

42. Pianezza ML, Sellers EM, Tyndale RF. Nicotine metabolism defect reduces smoking. Nature 1998; 393: 750.

43. Benowitz NL, Peres-Stable SJ, Herrera B, Jacob P. Slower metabolism and reduced intake of nicotine from cigarette smoking in Chinese-Americans. J Natl Cancer Inst 2002; 94: 108–115.

44. Zebetian CP, Gelernter J, Cubells JF. Functional variants at CYP2A6: new genotyping methods, population genetics, and relevance to studies of tobacco dependence. Am J Med Genet 2000; 96: 638–645.

45. Sellers EM, Kaplan HL, Tyndale RF. Inhibition of cytochrome P450 2A6 increases nicotine's oral bio-availability and decreases smoking. Clin Pharmacol Ther 2000; 68: 35–43.

46. Saarikoski ST, Sata F, Husgafvel-Pursiainen K, Rautalahti M. CYP2D6 ultrarapid metabolizer genotype as a potential modifier of smoking behaviour. Pharmacogenetics 2000; 10: 5–10.

47. Zevin S, Benowitz NL. Drug interactions with tobacco smoking. Clin Pharmakin 1999; 36: 425–438.

48. Upadhya SC, Tirumalai PS, Boyd MR et al. Cytochrome P4502E (CYP2E) in brain: constitutive expression, induction by ethanol and localisation by fluorescence in-situ hybridisation. Arch Biochem Biophys 2003: 373: 23–34.

49. Ingelman-Sundberg M, Johansson I, Yin H et al. Ethanol inducible cytochrome P4502E1: genetic polymorphism, regulation and possible role in the aetiology of alcohol-induced liver disease. Alcohol 1993; 10: 447–452.

50. Kharasch ED, Hankins DC, Cox K. Clinical isoflurane metabolism by cytochrome P450 2E1. Anaesthesiology 1999; 90: 766–771.

51. Kharasch ED, Thummel KE. Identification of cytochrome P450 2E1 as the predominant enzyme catalysing human liver microsomal defluorination of sevoflurane, isoflurane and methoxyflurane. Anaesthesiology 1993; 79: 795–807.

52. Sweeney BP. Why are smokers protected against PONV? Editorial: Br J Anaesthesiol 2002; 89: 1–4.

53. Mackenzie PL, Miners JO, McKinnon RA. Polymorphisms in UDP glucuronosyltransferase genes: functional consequences and clinical relevance. Clin Chem Lab Med 2000; 38: 889–892.

54. Cofman BL, King CD, Rios GR et al. The glucuronidation of opioids, other xenobiotics, and androgens by human UGT2B7Y and UGT2B7H. Drug Metab Dispos 1998; 26: 73–77.

55. Barbier O, Turgeon D, Girard C et al. 3-azido-3-deoxythymidine (AZT) is glucuronidated by human UDP-glucuronosyltransferase 2B7 (UGT2B7). Drug Metab Dispos 2000; 28: 497–502.

56. Cofman BL, Rios GR, King CD et al. Human UGT2B7 catalyses morphine glucuronidation. Drug Metab Dispos 1997; 25: 1–4.

57. Holthe M, Rakvag TN, Klepstad P et al. Sequence variation in the UDP-glucuronosyltransferase 2B7 (UGT2B7) gene: identification of 10 novel single nucleotide polymorphisms (SNPs) and analysis of their relevance to morphine glucuronidation in cancer patients. Pharmacogenomics J 2003; 3: 17–26.

58. Yates CR, Krynetski EY, Loennechen T. Molecular diagnosis of thiopurine S-methyltransferase deficiency: genetic basis for azathioprine and mercaptopurine intolerance. Ann Int Med 1997; 126: 608–614.

59. Schutz E, Gummert J, Mohr F. Azathioprine induced myelosupression in thiopurine methyltransferase deficient recipient. Lancet 1993; 341: 436.

60. McLeod HL, Relling MV, Liu Q et al. Polymorphic thiopurine methyltransferase in erythrocytes is indicative of activity in leukaemic blasts from children with acute lymphoblastic leukaemia. Blood 1995; 85: 1897–1902.

61. Tai HL, Krynetski EY, Schuetz EG et al. Enhanced proteolysis of thiopurine S-methyl transferase (TPMT) encoded by mutant alleles in humans (TPMT*2, TPMT*3). Mechanisms for the genetic polymorphisms of TPMT activity. Proc Natl Acad Sci USA 1997; 94: 6444–6449.

62. Evans WE, Han YY, Bomgars L et al. Preponderance of thiopurine S-methyltransferase deficiency and heterozygosity among patients intolerant to mercaptopurine or azathioprine. J Clin Oncol 2001; 19: 2293–2301.

63. Spielberg SP. N-acetyltransferases: pharmacogenetics and clinical consequences of polymorphic drug metabolism. J Pharmacokinet Biopharm 1996; 24: 509–519.

64. Grant DM, Meyer UA. Polymorphisms of N-acetyltransferase genes. Xenobiotica 1992; 22: 1073–1081.
65. Ilett KF, Kadlubar FF, Minchin RF. 1998 International meeting of the arylamine N-acetyltransferases: synopsis of the workshop on nomenclature, biochemistry, molecular biology, interspecies comparisons, and role in human disease risk. Drug Metab Dispos 1999; 27: 957–959.
66. Wikman H, Piirila P, Rosenberg C et al. N-acetyltransferase genotypes as modifiers of diisocyanate exposure-associated asthma risk. Pharmacogenetics 2002; 12: 227–233.
67. Lodish H, Berk A, Zipursky S. Transport across cell membranes. In: Molecular Cell Biology. New York: WH Freeman & Co., 2000; 578–615.
68. Yan Q. Pharmacogenomics of membrane transporters. In: Methods in Molecular Biology, vol. 227. Totowa, NJ: Humana Press Inc.
69. Hoffmeyer S, Burke O, von Richter O et al. Functional polymorphisms in the human-multidrug-resistance gene: multiple sequence variation and correlation of one allele with P-glycoprotein expression and activity *in vivo*. Proc Natl Acad Sci USA 2000; 97: 3473–3478.
70. Fromm MF, Eichelbaum M. The pharmacogenomics of human P-glycoprotein. In: Licinio J, Wong ML (eds) Pharmacogenomics: The Search for Individualised Therapies. Weinheim: Wiley-VCH Verlag, 2002; 159–175.
71. Kim RB. Drug transporters in HIV therapy. Top HIV Med 2003; 11: 136–139.
72. Choo EF, Leake B, Wandel C et al. Pharmacological inhibition of P-glycoprotein transport enhances the distribution of HIV-1 protease inhibitors into brain and testes. Drug Metab Dispos 2000; 28: 655–660.
73. Fellay J, Marzolini C, Meaden ER et al. Response to antiretroviral treatments in HIV-1 infected individuals with allelic variants of the multidrug resistance transporter 1: a pharmacogenetics study. Lancet 2002; 359: 30–36.
74. Hu M, Retz W, Baader M et al. Promoter polymorphism of the 5-HT transporter and Alzheimer's disease. Neurosci Lett 2000; 294: 63–65.
75. Sheppard DN, Welsh MJ. Structure and function of the CFTR chloride channel. Physiol Rev 1999; 79: S23–S45.
76. Caspi A, Sugden K, Moffitt TE et al. Influence of life stress on depression: moderation by a polymorphism in the 5-HTT gene. Science 2003; 301: 386–389.
77. Ho GT, Moodie FM, Satsangi J. Host bacterial interaction in the gut. Multidrug resistance 1 gene (P-glycoprotein 170): an important determinant in gastrointestinal disease? Gut 2003; 52: 759–766; [abstract].
78. Lin JJ, Yueh KC, Chang DC et al. The homozygote 10-copy genotype of variable number tandem repeat dopamine transporter gene may confer protection against Parkinson's disease for male, but not to female patients. J Neurol Sci 2003; 209: 87–92.
79. Liu S, Huang H, Lu X et al. Down regulation of thiamine transporter THTR2 gene expression in breast cancer and its association with resistance to apoptosis. Mol Cancer Res 2003; 1: 665–673.
80. Pendse S, Sayegh MH, Frank MII. P-glycoprotein – a novel therapeutic target for immunomodulation in clinical transplantation and autoimmunity? Curr Drug Target 2003; 4: 469–476.
81. Ma T, Thiagarajah JR, Yang H et al. Thiazolidinone CFTR inhibitor identified by high-throughput screening blocks cholera toxin-induced intestinal fluid secretion. J Clin Invest 2002; 110: 1651–1658.
82. Mansfield SG, Kole J, Puttaraju M et al. Repair of CFTR mRNA by spliceome-mediated RNA trans-splicing. Gene Ther 2000; 7: 1885–1895.

83. Bond C, LaForge KS, Tian M *et al*. Single nucleotide polymorphism in the human mu opioid receptor gene alters beta-endorphin binding and activity. Possible implications for opiate addiction. Proc Natl Acad Sci USA 1998; 95: 9608–9613.

84. Ongphiphadhanakul B, Chanprasertyothin S, Payatikul P *et al*. Oestrogen-receptor-alpha gene polymorphisms affect response in bone mineral density to oestrogen in post-menopausal women. Clin Endocrinol 2000; 52: 581–585.

85. Cohen BM, Ennulat DJ, Centorrino F *et al*. Polymorphisms of the dopamine D4 receptor and response to antipsychotic drugs. Psychopharmacology 1999; 141: 6–10.

86. Smeraldi E, Zenardi R, Benedetti F, Di Bella D. Polymorphisms within the promoter of the serotonin transporter gene and antidepressant efficacy of fluvoxamine. Mol Psychiatr 1998; 3: 508–511.

87. McCarthy TV, Quane KA, Lynch PJ. Ryanodine receptor mutations in malignant hyperthermia and central core disease. Hum Mutat 2000; 15: 410–417.

88. Ohmichi N, Iwai N, Uchida Y. Relationship between the response to the angiotensin converting enzyme inhibitor imidapril and the angiotensin converting enzyme genotype. Am J Hypertens 1997: 10: 951–955.

89. Iwai N, Ohmichi N, Nakamura Y. DD genotype of the angiotensin converting enzyme gene is a factor for left ventricular hypertrophy. Circulation 1994; 90: 2622–2628.

90. Aziz I, Hall IP, McFarlane LC *et al*. Beta-2-adrenoceptor regulation and bronchodilator sensitivity after regular treatment with formoterol in subjects with stable asthma. J Aller Clin Immunol 1998; 101: 337–341.

91. Weir TD, Mallek N, Sandford AJ *et al*. Beta2-adrenergic receptor haplotypes in mild, moderate, and fatal/near fatal asthma. Am J Respir Crit Care Med 1993; 158: 787–791.

92. Martinez FD, Graves PE, Baldini M *et al*. Association between genetic polymorphisms of the beta-2-adrenoceptor and response to albuterol in children with and without a history of wheezing. J Clin Invest 1997; 100: 3184–3188.

93. In KH, Asano K, Beier D *et al*. Naturally occurring mutations in the human 5-lipoxygenase gene promoter that modify transcription factor binding and reporter gene transcription. J Clin Invest 1997; 99: 1130–1137.

94. Drazen JM, Yandava CN, Dube L *et al*. Pharmacogenetic association between ALOX5 promoter genotype and the response to anti-asthma treatment. Nat Genet 1999; 22: 168–170.

95. Hansen T, Echwald SM, Hansen L *et al*. Decreased tolbutamide-stimulated insulin secretion in healthy subjects with sequence variants in the high-affinity sulfonylurea receptor gene. Diabetes 1998; 47: 598–605.

96. Cichon S, Nöthen MM, Rietsche M *et al*. Pharmacogenetics of schizophrenia. Am J Med Gen 2000; 97: 98–106.

97. Farlow MR, Lahiri DK, Poirier J *et al*. Treatment outcome of tacrine therapy depends upon apolipoprotein genotype and gender of the subjects. Neurology 1998; 50: 669–677.

98. Chen S, Zhang L, Bryant RM *et al*. KCNQ1 mutations in patients with a family history of lethal cardiac arrythmias and sudden death. Clin Genet 2003; 63: 273–282.

99. Eisen JA, Fraser CM. Phylogenomics: intersection of evolution and genomics. Science 2003; 300: 1706–1707.

100. Searls DB. Pharmacophylogenomics: genes, evolution and drug targets. Nature reviews. Drug Discovery 2003; 2: 613–623.

101. Witzman FA, Grant RA. Pharmacoproteomics in drug development. Pharmacogenomics J 2003; 2: 69–76.
102. Velculescu VE, Madden SL, Zhang Z. Analysis of human transcriptomes. Nat Genetics 1999; 23: 387–388.
103. Nuwaysir EF, Bittner M, Trent J *et al*. Microarrays and toxicology: the advent of toxicogenomics. Molec Carcinogen 1999; 24: 153–159.
104. Tefferi A, Bolander ME, Ansell SM *et al*. Primer on medical genomics. Pt III: microarray experiments and data analysis. Mayo Clin Proc 2002; 77: 927–940.
105. Zhang L, Zhou W, Velculescu VE *et al*. Gene expression profiles in normal and cancer cells. Science 1997; 276: 1268–1272.
106. Alizadeh AA, Eisen MB, Davis RE *et al*. Distinct type of diffuse large B-cell lymphoma identified by gene expression profiling. Nature 2000; 403: 503–511.
107. Cobb JP, Laramie JM, Stormo GD *et al*. Sepsis gene expression profiling: murine splenic compared with hepatic responses determined by using complementary DNA microarrays. Crit Care Med 2002; 30: 2711–2721.
108. Kozal MJ, Shah N, Shen N *et al*. Extensive polymorphisms observed in HIV-1 clade B protease gene using high density oligonucleotide arrays. Nat Med 1996; 2: 753–759.
109. Kaminsky N, Allard JD, Pittet JF *et al*. Global analysis of gene expression in pulmonary fibrosis reveals distinct programs regulating lung inflammation and fibrosis. Proc Natl Acad Sci USA 2000; 97: 1778–1783.
110. Stanton LW, Garrard LJ, Damm D *et al*. Altered patterns of gene expression in response to myocardial infarction. Circ Res 2000; 86: 161–172.
111. Marshall E. First check my genome doctor. Science 2003; 302: 589.
112. Stumm G, Russ A, Nehls M. Deductive genomics. A functional approach to identify innovative drug targets in the post-genomic era. Am J Pharmacogenet 2002; 2: 263–271.
113. Mcmanus TM, Sharp PA. Gene silencing in mammals by small interfering RNAs. Nature Rev Genet 2002; 3: 737–747.
114. Lapham EV, Kozma C, Weiss JO *et al*. Genetic discrimination: perspectives of consumers. Science 1996; 274: 621–624.
115. Pokorski RJ. Insurance underwriting in the genetic era. Am J Hum Gen 1997; 60: 205–221.
116. Lipton P. Pharmacogenetics: the ethical issues. Pharmacogenet J 2003; 3: 14–16.
117. Kanzok SM, Zheng L. The mosquito genome – a turning point? Trend Parasitol 2003; 19: 329–331.
118. Waxman DJ. P450 gene induction by structurally diverse xenochemicals: central role of nuclear receptors CAR, PXR and PPAR. Arch Biochem Biophys 1999; 369: 11–23.
119. Drews J, Ryser S. The role of innovation in drug development. Nature Biotechnol 1997; 15: 1318–1319.

Appendix: a compendium of interesting web sites related to pharmacogenomics

1. www.nuffieldbioethics.org – The Nuffield Council on Bioethics is the principle body in the UK dealing with ethical issues relating to pharmacogenomics research.

2. www.ebi.ac.uk/embl/index – The European Molecular Biology website has a number of interesting pages including a short tutorial on the latest aspects of bioinformatics and microarray technology.
3. www.ncbi.nlm.nih.gov – Centre for Biotechnology Information (NCBI) A comprehensive website which covers every aspect of molecular biology and genomic research. The website has an extremely useful search facility as well as educational pages and access to a map of the genomes of every organism which has been mapped so far.
4. www.ddbj.nig.ac.jp – DNA databank of Japan (DDBJ).
5. www.imm.ki.se/CYPalleles – A fully updated list of CYP enzymes together with a comprehensive list of their substrates and respective alleles can be found here.
6. www.gene.ucl.ac.uk/nomenclature/genefamily/abc.html – The Hugo Gene nomenclature website. A useful site for finding the names of genes.
7. www.ensembl.org/ – The home pages of Ensemble, a joint venture between the Sanger Trust and EMBL-EBI.
8. www.tigr.org – The Institute for Genome Research. Interesting information on plant genomes.
9. www.genome.gov/PolicyEthics/ – The National Human Genome Research Institute. A number of ethical and legislative issues are discussed here.

C. Zöllner   C. Stein

CHAPTER 2

The opioid receptor and opioid peptides

History

The opiates comprise a class of drugs also known as narcotic analgesics. Their principal effect is pain reduction. In addition, opiates produce a broad spectrum of side effects, including euphoria, that have lead to non-medicinal opiate use. Opioid use in history has been documented by ancient writings and archaeological data. The Sumerians cultivated poppies and isolated opium by drying and powdering the milky juice taken from the seed capsules of the opium poppy, *Papaver somniferum*. Opium was administered as a vapour, orally, or given through punctures in the skin. Due to the extreme variability in opium content and its variable rate of absorption, the effects varied from inadequate analgesia to respiratory depression and death. In 1806, the German chemist Sertürner isolated the most important alkaloid of opium, morphine, and named it after the god of dreams, Morpheus.[1] Opium consists of more than 25 alkaloids, including morphine (10%), codeine (0.5%), thebaine (0.3%), and papaverine (1%).[2] The effects of morphine were more potent and significantly more predictable than those of opium. The problem of accurate administration persisted until 1853, when Pravaz invented the syringe and Alexander Wood developed the hollow needle.[3] This development made more precise dosing possible and morphine began to be used for surgical procedures, for postoperative and chronic pain.

Structure and Activity

Although the alkaloid morphine was isolated in the early 1800s the structure of morphine was identified only in 1925 by Gullard and Robinson

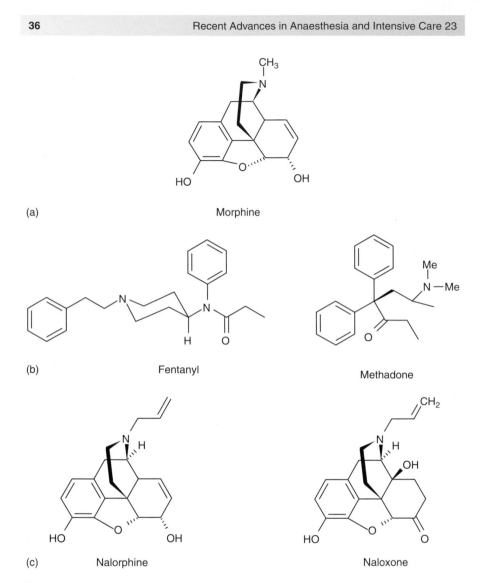

(a)   Morphine

(b)   Fentanyl

Methadone

(c)   Nalorphine   Naloxone

Figure 2.1 Structure of classical opioid receptor agonists (a) morphine; (b) 4-phenyl-piperidines (e.g. fentanyl) and the diphenylpropylamines (e.g. methadone); and opioid receptor antagonists (c) nalorphine and naloxone.

(Fig. 2.1a). From the structure of morphine it was hypothesized that the piperidine ring is essential for the pharmacological activity of the drug. The nitrogen atom of this ring is normally positively charged which can interact with a negatively charged counterpart. It was shown that simple modifications of the morphine molecule produce great variations in pharmacological potency. The addition of two acetyl groups in 1898 lead to the compound diacetylmorphine, or heroin, which was pronounced to be free from abuse liability. However, it was shown later that heroin is converted in the brain to monoacetylmorphine and then to morphine. The drug has a faster onset of action because the diacetylation increases lipid solubility and increases the passage through the blood–brain barrier. This was the first of many such claims to have produced more potent synthetic opioids with more potent analgesic activity and less physical and psychological dependence. However, despite tremendous efforts, to date only a few substances have been introduced into clinical practice. The 4-phenylpiperidines (e.g. fentanyl) and the diphenylpropylamines (e.g. methadone) were described as opiates with different structures from that of morphine (Fig. 2.1b). These compounds produce potent analgesia. However, they also produce side effects such as respiratory depression, reduced gastrointestinal motility, physical dependence and tolerance. In 1942 the substitution of an allyl group for the methyl group on the nitrogen atom of morphine produced the first opioid receptor antagonist, nalorphine. It was shown that nalorphine not only countered the effects of morphine but also produced limited analgesia mediated through κ-opioid receptors. This group of drugs was named mixed agonist–antagonists. Naloxone was developed as a relatively pure opioid receptor antagonist, which has a structure similar to that of morphine but cannot produce opioid-specific pharmacological agonist activity (Fig. 2.1c).

Opioid Receptors

Opioid receptor types

In the early 1970s it became evident, from classic dose–response curves and agonist–antagonist interactions, that several subtypes of opioid receptor existed:[4,5] μ, which is stimulated by morphine; δ, which binds the enkephalin analogue DPDPE ([D-penicillamine 2,5] enkephalin); and κ, which binds ketocyclazocine. The sigma receptor was initially described as an opioid receptor, for which the experimental compound SKF-10,047 had a high affinity. However, later it was not considered as an opioid receptor because it binds antipsychotic drugs such as haloperidol.[6]

Molecular cloning of opioid receptor types

The cloning of three different opioid receptor types had tremendous impact on our knowledge of gene and protein structure, opioid receptor function and regulation. The first opioid receptor was cloned almost simultaneously by two independent laboratories.[7,8] The cDNA was identified by expression cloning in mammalian cells. The protein, when expressed in transfected cells, showed the expected pharmacological profile of the δ-opioid receptor and is composed of 372 amino acid residues.

In addition, the protein showed structural characteristics similar to the family of seven transmembrane (TM) G-protein-coupled receptors. Subsequently, the μ-opioid receptor encoding a protein of 398 amino acids, and the κ-opioid receptor encoding a protein with 380 amino acid residues were cloned.[9,10] Classical pharmacological data during the past 30 years had suggested the concept of multiple receptor subtypes within each μ-, δ-, and κ-opioid receptor class. However, only three opioid receptor genes have been characterized so far and the issue of functional opioid receptor diversity remains controversial. Molecular mechanisms, which might explain the opioid receptor diversity, include alternative splicing from the known genes, post-translational modifications, association with distinct sets of G-proteins or cellular compartmentalization.[11]

Another opioid receptor cDNA with high sequence homology to the three cloned opioid receptors was isolated. The cDNA was named opioid-like orphan receptor 1 (ORL-1) due to its high homology and its G-protein-coupled receptor signalling system. However, a specific opioid-binding site to the ORL-1 receptor was not detectable. The opioid peptides show either relatively low affinity or no affinity toward the ORL-1 receptor. However, it was shown recently that the mutation of only four amino acids in the ORL-1 can produce a receptor that recognizes pro-dynorphin (PDYN) with high affinity and still binds the endogenous ORL-1 ligand.[12] This ligand was isolated by two groups.[13,14] The ligand was called orphanin FQ or nociceptin, which showed structural similarities to opioid peptides but did not bind at opioid receptors. In contrast to opioids, the supraspinal administration of nociceptin produces hyperalgesia. Spinal intrathecal and peripheral administration of nociceptin causes hyperalgesia in low doses and analgesia in high doses.[15] The mechanisms underlying the opposing directions of these nociceptive behaviours at different doses remain to be elucidated. In addition, nociceptin modulates other biological functions like feeding, locomotion, gastrointestinal function, memory, cardiovascular function, immunity, renal function, anxiety, dependence and tolerance. The diverse responses remain to be fully characterized before the compound can become a potential therapeutic target.[16,17]

Structural features of opioid receptors

Opioid receptors belong to the family of seven TM domain receptors. Seven membrane spanning domains are typical for receptors that are coupled to G-proteins. A sequence comparison between members of the opioid receptor family shows high similarity in TM 2, 3, 5, 6 and 7, the three intracellular loops, and a short region of the C-terminal tail. Figure 2.2

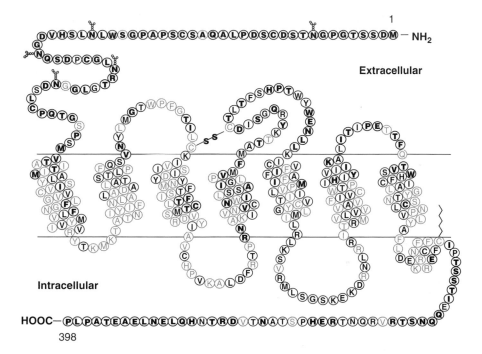

Figure 2.2 μ-opioid receptor topology. The seven α-helical TM domains characteristic of the μ-opioid receptor. Extracellular regions are above the TM domains, and include consensus sites for asparagine (N-linked) glycosylation (black forks) in the N-terminal tail. Bold letters: amino acid residues not shared with δ- and κ-opioid receptors. Black letters: residues common to all three opioid receptors. Grey letters: residues common to selected neuropeptide (e.g. somatostatin) and all three opioid receptors.

illustrates the putative TM topology of the rat μ-opioid receptor. Each amino acid residue is shown as a circle. Extracellular regions are above the TM domains, and include consensus sites for asparagine (N-linked) glycosylation (black forks) in the N-terminal tail. Bold letters represent amino acid residues not shared with δ- and κ-opioid receptors. Black letters represent residues common to all three opioid receptors. Grey letters represent residues common to selected neuropeptide (e.g. somatostatin) receptors and all three opioid receptors (Fig. 2.2). Almost no homology is found in the extracellular loops or in the N- and C-terminal tails of the receptors. The extracellular loops probably act as filters for the ligands and regulate the ability of the ligands to interact with the binding pocket.[18] No high-resolution structure of a human G-protein-coupled receptor has been resolved yet. This is mainly due to difficulties in obtaining large quantities of pure and active protein. Until now, only a high-resolution X-ray structure of an inactive state of bovine rhodopsin (another typical seven TM G-protein-coupled receptor) is available.[19] Structural motives, important for ligand binding and subtype specificity, can therefore only be predicted from experimental mutagenesis studies and computer modelling. These experiments have shown that the seven-helical bundle forms an opioid-binding pocket in which hydrophilic and aromatic residues from TM 2, 3, 6, and 7 contribute to ligand binding. Agonist binding to G-protein-coupled receptors is believed to promote a conformational change that leads to the formation of the active receptor state that will ultimately result in G-protein coupling and signal transduction.[20] Cysteine mutagenesis studies and computer modelling have indicated that movements of TM segments 3 and 6 are involved in activation of opioid receptors.[21,22] However, the mutation of single amino acids could affect the amino acid side-chain interaction and subsequently the tertiary structure of opioid receptors and does not allow the definitive identification of the binding sites. Intracellular domains are important for receptor signalling and regulation. The C-terminal portion of the receptor was shown to be important for receptor desensitization. A splice variant of the μ-opioid receptor, which differs only in length and amino acid composition at the very end of the C-terminal tail shows much more resistance to agonist-induced desensitization than the wild-type μ-opioid receptor construct.[23] In addition, the C-terminal part and the third intracellular loop seem to be involved in receptor trafficking (i.e. movement between membrane and intracellular compartments) and downregulation (i.e. reduction in receptor number). The mutation of the μ-opioid receptor at the C-terminal affected morphine-induced internalization without changing the relative agonist activity.[24]

Cellular Mechanisms of Action

Signal transduction

Opioids reduce the membrane excitability of neurones with subsequent slowing of cell firing and the inhibition of neurotransmitter release. The signalling pathways have been well characterized. After the ligand binds at the receptor, conformational changes allow coupling of mainly $G_{i/o}$-proteins to the opioid receptor. Dissociation of the trimeric G-protein complex into G_α and $G_{\beta\gamma}$ subunits can subsequently lead to inhibition of cyclic 3′5′ adenylyl cyclase (cyclic adenosine monophosphate, cAMP), to decrease in the conductance of voltage-gated Ca^{2+} channels or to the opening of rectifying K^+ channels (Fig. 2.3). cAMP might also be involved in long-term regulation of opioid neuropeptide synthesis.[25] cAMP-dependent protein kinase (PK) phosphorylates and activates cAMP-response element-binding proteins (CREB). CREB binds to specific DNA sequences in the promoter regions of genes and increases the mRNA synthesis for opioid (and other) neuropeptides. Opioid inhibition of adenylyl cyclase reduces the opioid peptide synthesis and represents a negative feedback in which high concentrations

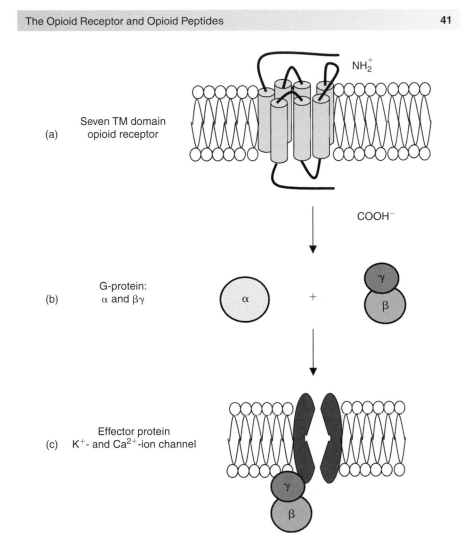

Figure 2.3 (a) Opioid ligands bind at the opioid receptor, inducing a conformational change at the receptor which allows coupling of G-proteins to the receptor. (b) Dissociation of the heterotrimeric G-protein into active G_α and $G_{\beta\gamma}$ subunits. (c) Active G_α and $G_{\beta\gamma}$ subunits can subsequently inhibit adenylyl cyclase, decrease the conductance of voltage-gated Ca^{2+} channels or open rectifying K^+ channels.

of endogenous peptides inhibit further cAMP-induced opioid neuropeptide synthesis.[25] Possibly via direct G-protein interactions, opioids directly close N-type and T-type Ca^{2+} channels and suppress pro-nociceptive neurotransmitter release in many neuronal systems.[26] A prominent example is the inhibition of substance P release from primary afferent sensory neurones in the spinal cord and from their peripheral terminals.[27] At the postsynaptic membrane (e.g. in the spinal cord), opioid receptors produce hyperpolarization by activating K^+ channels, thereby preventing excitation or propagation of action potentials. Apart from Ca^{2+} and K^+ channels opioid receptors may regulate the functions of other ion channels. For example, excitatory postsynaptic currents evoked by N-methyl-D-aspartate (NMDA) receptors or tetrodotoxin-resistant Na^+ channels in primary sensory neurones are inhibited by high concentrations of μ-opioid receptor agonists. Opioids block the channel at the same site where Mg^{2+} and ketamine can interfere with the NMDA receptor. This might be important under certain clinical conditions after epidural or intrathecal administration of opioids, where micromolar levels of the drug can be achieved in the spinal cord.[28]

Opioid receptor trafficking

The prolonged activation of opioid receptors leads to the expression of compensating mechanisms in many neurones or neuronal systems. Opioid receptor desensitization occurs as a consequence of G-protein uncoupling in response to phosphorylation by both second messenger-dependent protein kinases A and C (PKA and PKC, respectively) and G-protein-coupled receptor kinases (GRKs). GRK-mediated receptor phosphorylation promotes the binding of β-arrestins, which not only uncouple receptors from heterotrimeric G-proteins but also target many opioid receptors for internalization in clathrin-coated vesicles.[29,30] This process occurs after a few minutes of agonist exposure. Internalized receptors are either recycled to the cell surface after dephosphorylation or degraded in lysosomes (downregulation, i.e. reduction in the total number of receptors). Classically, receptor endocytosis has been thought to contribute directly to tolerance by decreasing the number of opioid receptors on the cell surface through the processes of desensitization and downregulation. Functional deletion of the β-arrestin 2 gene in mice resulted in remarkable potentiation and prolongation of the analgesic effect of opioids, indicating that the deletion of β-arrestin 2 can impair μ-opioid receptor desensitization and the development of tolerance.[31] However, studies indicate that certain opioid drugs such as morphine are deficient in their ability to induce the desensitization and endocytosis of receptors *in vivo* as well as in *in vitro* experiments.[32,33] It was shown that tolerance and withdrawal from morphine can decrease under conditions where receptors are trafficked through the endocytic and recycling pathway.[24] This finding suggests that acute desensitization might be a protective mechanism and prevents the development of tolerance. Drugs that do not cause receptor internalization, such as morphine, may have a higher propensity to develop tolerance. This might contribute to explain one of the fundamental questions in addiction biology, namely why exogenous opioid drugs have a high liability for inducing tolerance while native ligands do not. However, it is still unclear and under extensive controversial discussion whether these processes contribute to the acute or long-term changes in receptor sensitivity that occur after repeated exposure to opioids. Other neuroadaptations resulting from chronic opioid use include upregulation of the cAMP pathway, an increase in CREB protein and Fos-related antigens.[34] However, the connection between upregulation of these cellular elements and the mechanism behind the behavioural phenomenon remains unclear.[35] *In vivo* animal experiments have shown that tolerance development can be counteracted by NMDA antagonists.[36] These findings suggest that the combination of NMDA receptor antagonists with opioid analgesics might increase analgesic potency and prevent opioid-induced tolerance.[37] Clinically, tolerance is not ubiquitously observed and is in many cases explained by increasing nociceptive stimulation with progressing disease.[38] Similarly, animal models of pathological situations have also produced evidence for a reversal of tolerance to morphine during acute intestinal inflammation.[39] These findings indicate a potential for differences in opioid receptor desensitization and recycling under pathological situations and highlight the importance of studying animal models of persistent pain.

Opioid Ligands

Endogenous ligands

A fundamental finding in this field was that analgesia produced by electrically stimulating specific areas of the central nervous system could be partially antagonized by naloxone.[40] It was reasonable to consider that the stimulation-induced release of a natural ligand at the opioid receptor might be responsible. In 1974 a peptide in brain extracts was isolated that mimicked opioid activity and activated opioid receptors.[41] The isolated peptides were sequenced and identified as endogenous opioids, called endorphins from endo- signifying 'endogenous' and -orphin from the common suffix in the names of opioids. The endorphins are structurally related to pentapeptides. Two isoforms were identified first: Met-enkephalin (Tyr–Gly–Gly–Phe–Met) and Leu-enkephalin (Tyr–Gly–Gly–Phe–Leu).[41] Two additional peptides, β-endorphin and dypnorphin A, were identified later. The peptides were isolated from brain, pituitary gland, adrenals, immune cells, and other tissues. In addition, the spinal cord dorsal horn is rich in enkephalinergic and dynorphinergic neurones. These include terminals of primary afferents, spinal interneurones, and projection neurones. Noxious stimuli can release these opioids (particularly enkephalins) which have been suggested to act on primary afferent autoreceptors and postsynaptically. The N-terminal of all opioid peptides contains the Tyr–Gly–Gly–Phe–[Met/Leu] sequence followed by various C-terminal extensions. It was shown that three distinct opioid precursors exist: PDYN, pro-opiomelanocortin (POMC), and pro-enkephalin (PENK).[42–44] Each of the precursors must undergo processing by proteolytic enzymes into active fragments. The gene that codes for POMC is transcribed into mRNA that is translated into a prohormone of 267 amino acids. Post-translational processing of the large precursor peptide produces several smaller opioid peptides, including β-endorphin, α-melanocyte stimulating hormone (MSH), and adrenocorticotropic hormone (ACTH). Since these peptides play an important part in the body's response to stress, POMC could be a link between pain regulation and the stress response. The PENK gene encodes a protein precursor with 267 amino acids. Post-translational processing results in Met-enkephalin, Leu-enkephalin, and a number of enkephalin fragments, in particular bovine adrenal medulla peptide 22 (BAM22). A newly identified family of orphan G-protein-coupled receptors was cloned recently which bind BAM22 with nanomolar affinities. This family of receptors is uniquely localized in the human and rat small sensory neurones and was therefore called small sized sensory neurone-specific G-protein-coupled receptor (SNSR). Receptors of the SNSR family are distinct from the traditional opioid receptors in their insensitivity to the classical opioid antagonist naloxone and poor activation by opioid ligands. However, the unique localization of SNSRs and their activation by PENK A peptide fragments indicate a possible function for SNSRs in sensory neurone regulation and in the modulation of nociception.[45] The PDYN gene produces a prohormone of 254 amino acids, which encodes the opioid peptides dynorphin A and B, and α-neoendorphin.[46] So far, no obvious correspondence between any endogenous opioid peptide and a particular opioid receptor has been discovered. Each of the peptides can bind to any of the known opioid receptors with varying affinities. However, the PENK products show a relative preference for δ-opioid receptor and PDYN products for κ-opioid receptors.[47] Recently, a novel family of endogenous opioid peptides has been discovered and termed endomorphins.[48] Endomorphin-1 (Tyr–Pro–Trp–Phe) and endomorphin-2 (Tyr–Pro–Phe–Phe) are tetrapeptides which bind to the μ-opioid receptor with high affinity. The endomorphins have been found unequally distributed in the brain, peripheral nervous system, and in immune cells. They can be released from neurones and axon terminals by depolarization. Although the endomorphins are enzymatically converted by endopeptidases the precursor peptides have not been detected yet.[49]

Exogenous opioid receptor agonists

The pharmaceutic industrial standard to which all other opioid analgesics are compared is morphine. Morphine binds mainly to μ-opioid receptors where all the other opioids (fentanyl, sufentanil, and remifentanil) commonly used in the clinical setting can bind. However, all three receptors can mediate analgesic effects. In addition, μ- and δ-opioid receptors mediate respiratory depression, sedation, constipation, reward, and euphoria. κ-opioid receptors mediate dysphoric, aversive, and diuretic effects.

Opioids that have reduced efficacy at opioid receptors or act in addition as antagonists at other receptors are called partial agonists or mixed agonist/antagonists. This class includes pentazocine, nalbuphine, butorphanol, and buprenorphine. Their analgesic effects result from a weak, competitive partial agonist action at μ-opioid receptors and a full agonist action at κ-opioid receptors. As analgesics they are much less potent than morphine. Specific κ-opioid receptor agonists produce analgesia with little or no respiratory depression but with psychotomimetic and dysphoric effects. There are a number of commercially available κ-opioid receptor partial agonists, the so-called agonist–antagonists or nalorphine-like opioids, which appear to have minimal effects on respiration. Opioid receptor antagonists bind at opioid receptors without the induction of G-protein coupling. Two major drugs in this group, naloxone and naltrexone, which are full antagonists at μ-, δ-, κ-opioid receptors, have been introduced into the clinical setting. They are generally used to treat opioid overdose and are capable of reversing virtually all of the deleterious and beneficial effects of the opioids.

Functional Effects of Opioids

Supraspinal and spinal sites

Various major brain regions containing opioid peptides and opioid receptors have been identified including the periaqueductal grey, the locus coeruleus, and the rostral ventral medulla.[50] All three opioid receptors are also present in the dorsal horn of the spinal cord, which is in another major area of opioid-induced analgesia. μ-, δ-, κ-opioid receptors are mainly located in the upper laminae, particularly the substantia gelatinosa (laminae II). In addition, δ-opioid receptors are also found in the deeper laminae of the dorsal horn and in the ventral horn.[51] Opioids produce analgesia by depressing neuronal firing. Presynaptically, opioids can inhibit Ca^{2+} influx and the subsequent release of glutamate and neuropeptides (e.g. substance P, calcitonin gene-related peptide) from primary afferent terminals. Postsynaptically, opioids hyperpolarize ascending projection neurones by increasing K^+ conductance. Respiratory depression is the most important supraspinally mediated side effect of opioids under clinical conditions. This is caused by direct inhibition of rhythm-generating respiratory neurones in the pre-Botzinger complex of the brainstem.[52] It was recently shown that interneurones in this area coexpress μ-opioid receptors and a subtype of the serotonin (5-hydroxytryptamine, 5-HT) receptor (5-HT$_4$). 5-HT$_4$ and μ-opioid receptor-mediated pathways are coexistent in these inspiratory neurones. Opioid induced effects through $G_{i/o}$ which induce a decrease in the cAMP levels might by reversed by 5-HT$_4$ which activates G_s-proteins and raises cAMP concentrations. Stimulation of 5-HT$_4$ receptors in neurones of the medullary respiratory centre can effectively counteract fentanyl-induced respiratory depression without compromising its antinociceptive potency.[53] Opioid-induced nausea and vomiting are also important clinical side effects. Opioids mediate nausea and vomiting by stimulating the chemoreceptor trigger zone in the area postrema. Pupillary constriction is related to opioid stimulation of the Edinger–Westphal nuclei in the brainstem. This effect can be detected even after extremely small doses of opioids and can therefore be used as a tool to evaluate drug effects. Excitatory side effects such as allodynia or hyperalgesia might be related to metabolites of morphine, which is degraded to morphine-3-glucoronide (M3G) and morphine-6-glucuronide (M6G). M6G is a compound with an even higher opioid activity than morphine. High concentrations of M3G can cause excitatory side effects which cannot be blocked by naloxone.

Peripheral sites

It became clear in the late 1980s that opioid receptors and opioid peptides are not only located in the central but also in the peripheral nervous system, including primary afferent neurones and dorsal root ganglia.[54] All three opioid receptors have been shown mainly on small-to-medium diameter neuronal cell bodies of sensory neurones.[55] After synthesis, opioid receptors are transported to the central as well as peripheral nerve terminals of primary afferent neurones.[56] Opioid receptors are also expressed by neuroendocrine (pituitary, adrenals), immune, and ectodermal tissues.[57] Although opioids increase K^+ currents in the central nervous system, it is still controversial whether this occurs in dorsal root ganglion neurones. Rather, it was shown that the modulation of Ca^{2+} currents is the principal mechanism for the inhibitory effect of opioids on sensory neurones.[58] However, G-protein-coupled inwardly rectifying K^+ (GIRK2) channels and μ-opioid receptors were recently colocalized on sensory nerve endings in rat plantar hind-paw epidermis and it was proposed that endothelin-B receptors trigger the release of endorphin from keratinocytes, suppressing pain via opioid receptors coupled to GIRK channels.[59] In addition, opioids can activate inhibitory $G_{i/o}$-proteins which lead to a decrease of cAMP in peripheral sensory neurones (Fig. 2.4).[60]

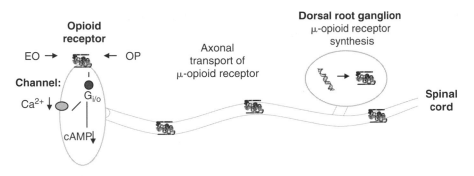

Figure 2.4 Opioid receptors are synthesized in the dorsal root ganglion and transported intra-axonally to the central and peripheral terminals of primary afferent neurones. Exogenous (EO) or endogenous (OP) opioids can activate the signal transduction cascade which leads to G-protein coupling, suppression of cAMP and a decrease of Ca^{2+} currents. Subsequently, this reduces excitability of the cell membrane and neurotransmitter release.

Peripheral opioid receptors and inflammation

In animal experiments it was shown that local application of μ-opioid receptor agonists elicits a more pronounced antinociceptive effect under painful inflammatory conditions than in non-inflamed tissue. Potential mechanisms for an increase in antinociception might involve an increase in the number of opioid receptors. It was shown that subcutaneous inflammation can induce an upregulation of μ-opioid receptor mRNA within the lumbar spinal cord.[61] In addition, the expression of opioid receptors in sensory neurones increases time dependently in similar models of painful inflammation.[62] Subsequently, the axonal transport of opioid receptors from sensory neurones to the peripheral nerve terminals is augmented and can be reduced by ligation of the sciatic nerve, indicating that subcutaneous inflammation enhances the peripherally directed axonal transport of opioid receptors.[63,64] This increase might be related to certain cytokines (e.g. interleukin 4) through the binding of signal transducer and activator of transcription factors (STAT: STAT-6) to the μ-opioid receptor gene promotor.[65] It was recently shown that the activation of mitogen-activated protein kinases (MAPKs: p38-MAPK) in dorsal root ganglion neurones following inflammation-induced retrograde intra-axonal transport of nerve growth factor (NGF) can increase the capsaicin sensitive transient receptor potential channel VR1 (TRPV1).[66] NGF might also be involved in μ-opioid receptor upregulation during inflammation. Other potential mechanisms, which might explain an increase in opioid antinociception under inflammation, include an increase in the number of opioid-receptor-bearing peripheral sensory nerve terminals.[27] In addition, exogenous opioids can lead to an increase in G-protein coupling.[62] Thus, neuronal opioid receptors in the inflamed paw might undergo changes owing to the specific milieu of inflamed tissue (e.g. low pH) which could contribute to an increase in opioid efficacy.[67] Finally, inflammation can also disrupt the perineurium which is normally a rather impermeable barrier. This allows exogenous opioid agonists easier access to peripheral opioid receptors. These adaptive changes underscore the important differences in opioid receptor binding and signalling between normal and inflamed tissue.

Inflammation and endogenous opioid peptides

The analgesic effects of endogenous opioids in painful inflammation can be blocked by antibodies against opioid peptides and by immunosuppression, suggesting the involvement of the immune system. The endogenous opioid peptides (mainly β-endorphin and met-enkephalin) as well as mRNA encoding POMC and PENK are present within lymphocytes, monocytes, and granulocytes in inflamed tissue.[68] In models of inflammatory pain, opioid peptide-containing immune cells migrate from the circulation to the injured tissue. Selectins have been identified as important adhesion molecules which regulate the migration of opioid peptide-containing immune cells.[69] Upon certain exogenous stressful stimuli (e.g. cold water swim stress or postoperative pain), these cells can locally release opioid peptides which subsequently bind to opioid receptors on sensory neurones, where they can increase the nociceptive thresholds. In humans, the intra-articular application of naloxone after knee arthroscopy can increase pain in the presence of endogenous opioid peptides within synovial tissue. These studies have suggested that a stressful stimulus (e.g. surgery) leads to a tonic release of endogenous opioids to reduce inflammatory pain by activating intra-articular opioid receptors.[70] Opioid-containing cells are predominantly granulocytes during early and monocytes or macrophages during later stages of inflammation.[68] The endogenous opioid-mediated analgesia increases in parallel with the immune cell recruitment and the degree of inflammation. Other endogenous stimuli have been identified to trigger opioid secretion from immune cells. For instance, corticotropin-releasing hormone (CRH) stimulates the release of opioid peptides from immune cells which subsequently activate opioid receptors on sensory nerve endings.[71] These results indicate that the activation of the endogenous opioid production and the release from immune cells might be an innovative strategy for the development of novel peripherally acting analgesics.

Peripheral opioids and clinical implications

Since the first demonstration of the analgesic efficacy of intra-articular morphine, many clinical and experimental studies confirmed that application of peripheral opioids in patients or animals with acute and chronic pain results in significant pain reduction. In dental surgery peripheral antinociception was detected after local morphine application.[27,72] In patients with chronic arthritis the effects of local morphine has also been shown to reduce pain.[73] The intra-articular injection of morphine can produce a long-lasting analgesia of up to 6 days. However, it was shown that the three major opioid receptor types are differentially expressed in peripheral tissues, indicating that different opioid agonists might not be equally effective. In rat paw skin, all three receptor types have been reported to be functionally active.[54] In contrast, only κ-opioid receptor ligands are effective in attenuating visceral nociceptor activity.[74] Clinical studies have shown that topical application of opioids produces significant antihyperalgesic effects when applied to painful ulcers and skin lesions, after burn injuries and in cutaneous pain in a palliative care setting.[75–78] The local application of morphine in patients with corneal abrasion also showed strong analgesic effects.[79] Current studies are investigating whether opioids might be beneficial in patients with chronic arthritic pain with particular attention to the possible anti-inflammatory effects of peripheral opioids.[73] Two novel peripherally restricted κ-opioid peptides with potent analgesic and anti-inflammatory properties have been recently investigated and may lead to improved analgesic therapy compared with centrally acting opioids or standard non-steroidal anti-inflammatory drugs.[80] In many of these studies peripheral analgesic effects were shown to be dose-dependent and reversible by naloxone, indicating specific opioid receptor-mediated effects. In addition, studies have shown that relatively little analgesic tolerance develops after repeated administration of peripheral opioid agonists in inflamed tissue.[81]

Summary

Considering that the local route of administration is easy and carries only minimal risks of side effects, these findings could stimulate new approaches to opioid therapy for many other pain-related diseases. The absence of central side effects opens new possibilities for acute and chronic pain therapy. New approaches to increase the synthesis or secretion of peripheral endogenous opioid peptides such as vectors containing PENK cDNA, gene-gun systems with POMC, cDNA or chemokines that attract opioid-producing cells to damaged tissue could open exciting possibilities for pain research and therapy in the future.[82]

References

1. Schmitz R. Friedrich Wilhelm Sertürner and the discovery of morphine. Pharm Hist 1985; 27: 61–74.
2. Hosztafi S. The discovery of alkaloids. Pharmazie 1997; 52: 546–550.
3. Musto DF. Opium, cocaine and marijuana in American history. Sci Am 1991; 265: 40–47.

4. Pert CB, Snyder SH. Opiate receptor: demonstration in nervous tissue. Science 1973; 179: 1011–1014.

5. Martin WR, Eades CG, Thompson JA, Huppler RE, Gilbert PE. The effects of morphine- and nalorphine-like drugs in the nondependent and morphine-dependent chronic spinal dog. J Pharmacol Exp Ther 1976; 197: 517–532.

6. Tam SW. Naloxone-inaccessible sigma receptor in rat central nervous system. Proc Natl Acad Sci USA 1983; 80: 6703–6707.

7. Evans CJ, Keith Jr, DE, Morrison H, Magendzo K, Edwards RH. Cloning of a delta opioid receptor by functional expression. Science 1992; 258: 1952–1955.

8. Kieffer B, Befort K, Gaveriaux-Ruff C, Hirth C. The d-opioid receptor: isolation of a cDNA by expression cloning and pharmacological characterization. Proc Natl Acad Sci USA 1992; 12048–12052.

9. Wang JB, Imai Y, Eppler CM, Gregor P, Spivak CE, Uhl GR. mu opiate receptor: cDNA cloning and expression. Proc Natl Acad Sci USA 1993; 90: 10230–10234.

10. Meng F, Xie GX, Thompson RC et al. Cloning and pharmacological characterization of a rat kappa opioid receptor. Proc Natl Acad Sci USA 1993; 90: 9954–9958.

11. Kieffer BL. Opioid receptors: gene structure and function. In: Stein C (ed.) Opioids in Pain Control. Cambridge: Cambridge University Press, 1999; 1–20.

12. Meng F, Taylor LP, Hoversten MT et al. Moving from the orphanin FQ receptor to an opioid receptor using four point mutations. J Biol Chem 1996; 271: 32016–32020.

13. Meunier JC, Mollereau C, Toll L et al. Isolation and structure of the endogenous agonist of opioid receptor-like ORL1 receptor. Nature 1995; 377: 532–535.

14. Reinscheid RK, Nothacker HP, Bourson A et al. Orphanin FQ: a neuropeptide that activates an opioid like G protein-coupled receptor. Science 1995; 270: 792–794.

15. Grond S, Meuser T, Pietruck C, Sablotzki A. [Nociceptin and the ORL1 receptor: pharmacology of a new opioid receptor]. Anaesthesist 2002; 51: 996–1005.

16. New DC, Wong YH. The ORL1 receptor: molecular pharmacology and signalling mechanisms. Neurosignals 2002; 11: 197–212.

17. Mogil JS, Pasternak GW. The molecular and behavioral pharmacology of the orphanin FQ/nociceptin peptide and receptor family. Pharmacol Rev 2001; 53: 381–415.

18. Law PY, Wong YH, Loh HH. Molecular mechanisms and regulation of opioid receptor signaling. Annu Rev Pharmacol Toxicol 2000; 40: 389–430.

19. Palczewski K, Kumasaka T, Hori T et al. Crystal structure of rhodopsin: a G protein-coupled receptor. Science 2000; 289: 739–745.

20. Gether U, Kobilka BK. G protein-coupled receptors. II. Mechanism of agonist activation. J Biol Chem 1998; 273: 17979–17982.

21. Gether U, Lin S, Ghanouni P, Ballesteros JA, Weinstein H, Kobilka BK. Agonists induce conformational changes in transmembrane domains III and VI of the beta2 adrenoceptor. EMBO J 1997; 16: 6737–6747.

22. Strahs D, Weinstein H. Comparative modeling and molecular dynamics studies of the delta, kappa and mu opioid receptors. Protein Eng 1997; 10: 1019–1038.

23. Zimprich A, Simon T, Hollt V. Cloning and expression of an isoform of the rat mu opioid receptor (rMOR1B) which differs in agonist induced desensitization from rMOR1. FEBS Lett 1995; 359: 142–146.

24. Whistler JL, Chuang HH, Chu P, Jan LY, von Zastrow M. Functional dissociation of mu opioid receptor signaling and endocytosis: implications for the biology of opiate tolerance and addiction. Neuron 1999; 23: 737–746.

25. Childers S. Opioid receptor-coupled second messenger systems. In: Herz A (ed.) Opioids I, Handbook of Experimental Pharmacology. New York: Springer Verlag, 1993; 189–216.

26. Dogrul A, Yesilyurt O, Isimer A, Guzeldemir ME. L-type and T-type calcium channel blockade potentiate the analgesic effects of morphine and selective mu opioid agonist, but not to selective delta and kappa agonist at the level of the spinal cord in mice. Pain 2001; 93: 61–68.

27. Stein C. The control of pain in peripheral tissue by opioids. New Engl J Med 1995; 332: 1685–1690.

28. Yamakura T, Sakimura K, Shimoji K. Direct inhibition of the N-methyl-D-aspartate receptor channel by high concentrations of opioids. Anesthesiology 1999; 91: 1053–1063.

29. Ferguson SS. Evolving concepts in G protein-coupled receptor endocytosis: the role in receptor desensitization and signaling. Pharmacol Rev 2001; 53: 1–24.

30. Whistler JL, von Zastrow M. Morphine-activated opioid receptors elude desensitization by beta-arrestin. Proc Natl Acad Sci USA 1998; 95: 9914–9919.

31. Bohn LM, Lefkowitz RJ, Gainetdinov RR, Peppel K, Caron MG, Lin FT. Enhanced morphine analgesia in mice lacking beta-arrestin 2. Science 1999; 286: 2495–2498.

32. Eisinger DA, Ammer H, Schulz R. Chronic morphine treatment inhibits opioid receptor desensitization and internalization. J Neurosci 2002; 22: 10192–10200.

33. Stafford K, Gomes AB, Shen J, Yoburn BC. mu-Opioid receptor downregulation contributes to opioid tolerance *in vivo*. Pharmacol Biochem Behav 2001; 69: 233–237.

34. Nestler EJ, Aghajanian GK. Molecular and cellular basis of addiction. Science 1997; 278: 58–63.

35. Borgland SL. Acute opioid receptor desensitization and tolerance: is there a link? Clin Exp Pharmacol Physiol 2001; 28: 147–154.

36. Elliott K, Kest B, Man A, Kao B, Inturrisi CE. N-methyl-D-aspartate (NMDA) receptors, mu and kappa opioid tolerance, and perspectives on new analgesic drug development. Neuropsychopharmacology 1995; 13: 347–356.

37. Price DD, Mayer DJ, Mao J, Caruso FS. NMDA-receptor antagonists and opioid receptor interactions as related to analgesia and tolerance. J Pain Symptom Manage 2000; 19: S7–S11.

38. Collett BJ. Opioid tolerance: the clinical perspective. Br J Anaesth 1998; 81: 58–68.

39. Pol O, Puig MM. Reversal of tolerance to the antitransit effects of morphine during acute intestinal inflammation in mice. Br J Pharmacol 1997; 122: 1216–1222.

40. Akil H, Mayer DJ, Liebeskind JC. Antagonism of stimulation-produced analgesia by naloxone, a narcotic antagonist. Science 1976; 191: 961–962.

41. Hughes J, Smith TW, Kosterlitz HW, Fothergill LA, Morgan BA, Morris HR. Identification of two related pentapeptides from the brain with potent opiate agonist activity. Nature 1975; 258: 577–580.

42. Kakidani H, Furutani Y, Takahashi H *et al*. Cloning and sequence analysis of cDNA for porcine beta-neo-endorphin/dynorphin precursor. Nature 1982; 298: 245–249.

43. Nakanishi S, Inoue A, Kita T *et al*. Nucleotide sequence of cloned cDNA for bovine corticotropin–beta-lipotropin precursor. Nature 1979; 278: 423–427.

44. Comb M, Seeburg PH, Adelman J, Eiden L, Herbert E. Primary structure of the human Met- and Leu-enkephalin precursor and its mRNA. Nature 1982; 295: 663–666.

45. Lembo PM, Grazzini E, Groblewski T et al. Proenkephalin A gene products activate a new family of sensory neuron – specific GPCRs. Nat Neurosci 2002; 5: 201–209.
46. Höllt V. Regulation of opioid peptide gene expression. In: Herz A (ed.) Opioids I, Handbook of Experimental Pharmacology. New York: Springer Verlag, 1993; 307–346.
47. Akil H, Owens C, Gutstein H, Taylor L, Curran E, Watson S. Endogenous opioids: overview and current issues. Drug Alcohol Depend 1998; 51: 127–140.
48. Zadina JE, Hackler L, Ge LJ, Kastin AJ. A potent and selective endogenous agonist for the mu-opiate receptor. Nature 1997; 386: 499–502.
49. Horvath G. Endomorphin-1 and endomorphin-2: pharmacology of the selective endogenous mu-opioid receptor agonists. Pharmacol Ther 2000; 88: 437–463.
50. Heinricher M, Morgan M. Supraspinal mechanisms of opioid analgesia. In: Stein C (ed.) Opioids in Pain Control: Basic and Clinical Aspects. Cambridge: Cambridge University Press, 1999; 46–69.
51. Gouarderes C, Tellez S, Tafani JA, Zajac JM. Quantitative autoradiographic mapping of delta-opioid receptors in the rat central nervous system using [125I][D.Ala2]deltorphin-I. Synapse 1993; 13: 231–240.
52. Smith JC, Ellenberger HH, Ballanyi K, Richter DW, Feldman JL. Pre-Botzinger complex: a brainstem region that may generate respiratory rhythm in mammals. Science 1991; 254: 726–729.
53. Manzke T, Guenther U, Ponimaskin EG et al. 5-HT4(a) receptors avert opioid-induced breathing depression without loss of analgesia. Science 2003; 301: 226–229.
54. Stein C, Millan MJ, Shippenberg TS, Peter K, Herz A. Peripheral opioid receptors mediating antinociception in inflammation. Evidence for involvement of mu, delta and kappa receptors. J Pharmacol Exp Ther 1989; 248: 1269–1275.
55. Mousa SA, Machelska H, Schafer M, Stein C. Co-expression of beta-endorphin with adhesion molecules in a model of inflammatory pain. J Neuroimmunol 2000; 108: 160–170.
56. Antonijevic I, Mousa SA, Schafer M, Stein C. Perineurial defect and peripheral opioid analgesia in inflammation. J Neurosci 1995; 15: 165–172.
57. Slominski A, Wortsman J, Luger T, Paus R, Solomon S. Corticotropin releasing hormone and proopiomelanocortin involvement in the cutaneous response to stress. Physiol Rev 2000; 80: 979–1020.
58. Akins PT, McCleskey EW. Characterization of potassium currents in adult rat sensory neurons and modulation by opioids and cyclic AMP. Neuroscience 1993; 56: 759–769.
59. Khodorova A, Navarro B, Jouaville LS et al. Endothelin-B receptor activation triggers an endogenous analgesic cascade at sites of peripheral injury. Nat Med 2003; 9: 1055–1061.
60. Chen JJ, Dymshitz J, Vasko MR. Regulation of opioid receptors in rat sensory neurons in culture. Mol Pharmacol 1997; 51: 666–673.
61. Maekawa K, Minami M, Masuda T, Satoh M. Expression of mu- and kappa-, but not delta-, opioid receptor mRNAs is enhanced in the spinal dorsal horn of the arthritic rats. Pain 1996; 64: 365–371.
62. Zollner C, Shaqura MA, Bopaiah CP, Mousa S, Stein C, Schafer M. Painful inflammation-induced increase in micro-opioid receptor binding and G-protein coupling in primary afferent neurons. Mol Pharmacol 2003; 64: 202–210.
63. Laduron PM, Castel MN. Axonal transport of receptors. A major criterion for presynaptic localization. Ann NY Acad Sci 1990; 604: 462–469.

64. Hassan AH, Ableitner A, Stein C, Herz A. Inflammation of the rat paw enhances axonal transport of opioid receptors in the sciatic nerve and increases their density in the inflamed tissue. Neuroscience 1993; 55: 185–195.

65. Kraus J, Borner C, Giannini E et al. Regulation of mu-opioid receptor gene transcription by interleukin-4 and influence of an allelic variation within a STAT6 transcription factor binding site. J Biol Chem 2001; 276: 43901–43908.

66. Ji RR, Samad TA, Jin SX, Schmoll R, Woolf CJ. p38 MAPK activation by NGF in primary sensory neurons after inflammation increases TRPV1 levels and maintains heat hyperalgesia. Neuron 2002; 36: 57–68.

67. Selley DE, Breivogel CS, Childers SR. Modification of G protein-coupled functions by low-pH pretreatment of membranes from NG108-15 cells: increase in opioid agonist efficacy by decreased inactivation of G proteins. Mol Pharmacol 1993; 44: 731–741.

68. Rittner HL, Brack A, Machelska H et al. Opioid peptide-expressing leukocytes: identification, recruitment, and simultaneously increasing inhibition of inflammatory pain. Anesthesiology 2001; 95: 500–508.

69. Machelska H, Mousa SA, Brack A et al. Opioid control of inflammatory pain regulated by intercellular adhesion molecule-1. J Neurosci 2002; 22: 5588–5596.

70. Stein C, Hassan AH, Lehrberger K, Giefing J, Yassouridis A. Local analgesic effect of endogenous opioid peptides. Lancet 1993; 342: 321–324.

71. Schafer M, Mousa SA, Stein C. Corticotropin-releasing factor in antinociception and inflammation. Eur J Pharmacol 1997; 323: 1–10.

72. Likar R, Sittl R, Gragger K et al. Peripheral morphine analgesia in dental surgery. Pain 1998; 76: 145–150.

73. Likar R, Schafer M, Paulak F et al. Intraarticular morphine analgesia in chronic pain patients with osteoarthritis. Anesth Analg 1997; 84: 1313–1317.

74. Burton MB, Gebhart GF. Effects of kappa-opioid receptor agonists on responses to colorectal distension in rats with and without acute colonic inflammation. J Pharmacol Exp Ther 1998; 285: 707–715.

75. Kolesnikov YA, Chereshnev I, Pasternak GW. Analgesic synergy between topical lidocaine and topical opioids. J Pharmacol Exp Ther 2000; 295: 546–551.

76. Twillman RK, Long TD, Cathers TA, Mueller DW. Treatment of painful skin ulcers with topical opioids. J Pain Symptom Manage 1999; 17: 288–292.

77. Long TD, Cathers TA, Twillman R, O'Donnell T, Garrigues N, Jones T. Morphine-infused silver sulfadiazine (MISS) cream for burn analgesia: a pilot study. J Burn Care Rehabil 2001; 22: 118–123.

78. Krajnik M, Zylicz Z, Finlay I, Luczak J, van Sorge AA. Potential uses of topical opioids in palliative care – report of 6 cases. Pain 1999; 80: 121–125.

79. Peyman GA, Rahimy MH, Fernandes ML. Effects of morphine on corneal sensitivity and epithelial wound healing: implications for topical ophthalmic analgesia. Br J Ophthalmol 1994; 78: 138–141.

80. Binder W, Machelska H, Mousa S et al. Analgesic and antiinflammatory effects of two novel kappa-opioid peptides. Anesthesiology 2001; 94: 1034–1044.

81. Stein C, Pfluger M, Yassouridis A et al. No tolerance to peripheral morphine analgesia in presence of opioid expression in inflamed synovia. J Clin Invest 1996; 98: 793–799.

82. Stein C, Schafer M, Machelska H. Attacking pain at its source: new perspectives on opioids. Nat Med 2003; 9: 1003–1008.

M. Laffan

Coagulation

The development of large organisms has necessitated the parallel development of a fluid transport system (blood) and a system to contain it (the vasculature). This then puts the organism at risk of death from haemorrhage and so a coagulation system is required to rapidly seal breaches of the vessel walls. Such a powerful mechanism is itself dangerous and without regulation may inappropriately occlude the vessels with equally fatal consequences. Thus, we come to live in an uneasy balance between haemorrhage and thrombosis. The effects of illness, surgery, pregnancy and eventually age all serve to make this balance more precarious. To manage this problem, we have evolved a complex system of amplification and regulation, which produces rapid and effective clot formation restricted to the appropriate site with additional fibrinolytic mechanisms to eventually remove the clot as part of the healing process. The safety of the coagulation system is founded on the retention of these highly potent and complex systems within the vasculature and keeping them separate from their co-factor triggers, which are positioned outside. Thus the system is only fired when the two meet following breach of the vessel walls. As is well known, the consequences of intravascular exposure of these triggers, which occurs in malignancy and sepsis, can be catastrophic.

This review will briefly describe the normal mechanism of coagulation before discussing the essential features and management, of hereditary and acquired disorders of coagulation.

Normal Haemostasis

Breach of the vessel wall results in exposure of two important molecular triggers for the coagulation system, tissue factor (TF) and collagen, which act in concert with the rapid flow of blood over the damaged vessel wall. The subsequent events are complex, simultaneous and interwoven but will be separated here for clarity.

Primary haemostasis

Initially, haemostasis is achieved by formation of a platelet plug.[1] Plasma von Willebrand factor (VWF) binds to collagen exposed beneath the damaged endothelium and is extended by the shear stress of the escaping blood from its circulating globular form into an elongated linear form of great length. The functional activity of VWF is critically dependent on its length, reflecting the formation of high-molecular-weight multimers. Some VWF, having been secreted in an abluminal fashion by the vascular endothelial cells, will already be bound to sub-endothelial collagen. Elongation of VWF exposes the multiple platelet binding sites. Platelets are first transiently captured, slowed and activated by the interaction between VWF and platelet glycoprotein Ib (GpIb). After release they are recaptured and released again, thus appearing to 'roll' along the VWF molecule.[2,3] GpIb binding-induced activation leads to a conformational change in platelet GpIIbIIIa which, when the platelet is slowed, is able to achieve secure tethering of the platelet to collagen (Fig. 3.1). Platelets also bind directly to collagen via GpIaIIa and GpVI, which contribute to activation and, at certain shear stresses, to capture.[2,3] Platelet activation also causes release of platelet granules containing many platelet-activating substances, in particular adenosine diphosphate (ADP), of further amounts of VWF, and synthesis and release of thromboxane.[4] This next layer of VWF captures more platelets, and so a plug of platelets accumulates, bound together by VWF with contributions also from fibrinogen and fibronectin. The platelet plug is sufficient on its own to complete haemostasis after small superficial injuries (hence the bleeding time is normal in haemophilia); however, larger injuries require the plug to be stabilized by fibrin.

Although there appears to be considerable redundancy in this system, not all participants are equal. Thus, the absence of GpIIbIIIa or VWF results in very severe bleeding disorders, but absence of IaIIa[5] or plasma fibronectin does not.[6] Defects of primary haemostasis are described below.

Coagulation (fibrin generation)

The function of the coagulation system is to generate thrombin, the multifunctional enzyme that converts soluble plasma fibrinogen into the insoluble

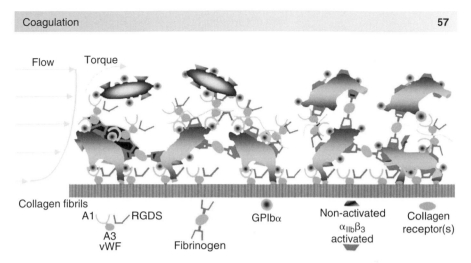

Flow Torque

Collagen fibrils
A1 RGDS
A3
vWF Fibrinogen GPIbα Non-activated Collagen
$\alpha_{IIb}\beta_3$ receptor(s)
activated

Figure 3.1 Schematic representation of the mechanisms of platelet adhesion and aggregation in flowing blood. In a cylindrical vessel, the velocity profile of particles contained in circulating blood is parabolic; the shear rate decreases from the wall to the centre of the lumen inversely to the flow velocity. In a flow field with high shear rate, only GPIb interaction with immobilized VWF multimers can initiate the tethering of circulating platelets to the vessel wall and to already adherent platelets. This GPIb-dependent interaction supports initially transient bonds, depicted by the ongoing detachment of the two top platelets from VWF multimers bound to already activated platelets. The process is amplified by the activation of $\alpha_{IIb}\beta_3$, which may occur during the transient tethering or through the action of other receptors that bind collagen or other components of exposed vascular or extravascular surfaces. The final result is stable attachment of recruited platelets and irreversible membrane binding of soluble adhesive ligand (fibrinogen and VWF), thus providing the substrate for additional recruitment of non-activated platelets and leading to thrombus growth. Note that non-activated $\alpha_{IIb}\beta_3$ cannot bind soluble ligands. The bridging effect of fibrinogen, which is required to stabilize platelet aggregation and resist the effects of high shear stress, only occurs after initial tethering of platelets through the interaction of VWF and GPIb. At shear rates <500–$1000\,s^{-1}$, the adhesive functions of VWF are no longer indispensable, either for initial attachment to a thrombogenic surface or for aggregation. Thus, even in the absence of VWF, collagen receptors (among others) can permit stable adhesive interactions to form rapidly, and fibrin or fibrinogen can bind to platelets to permit aggregation. Redrawn with permission from Zaverio and Ruggeri. J Clin Invest 2000; 105: 699–701.

fibrin clot. This process is triggered by the formation of the active TF–factor VIIa complex. Approximately 1% of plasma factor VII is already in its activated form (VIIa), but it is not functional as an enzyme until it is complexed with TF.[7] TF is a transmembrane receptor expressed widely throughout the body on many cells including fibroblasts and myocytes but not normally within the vasculature. As coagulation is only initiated when TF and VIIa meet, the system is not activated until a vessel wall is breached. Thus, TF is said to form a 'haemostatic envelope' around the vasculature.[8]

The TF–VIIa complex initiates coagulation by specific proteolytic cleavage of factors X and IX, converting them to their active forms, factors Xa and IXa, respectively. The factor Xa so formed is able to cleave a small amount of prothrombin into thrombin on the surface of the TF-bearing cell.[9] This mechanism alone does not generate sufficient thrombin for effective haemostasis, and is rapidly extinguished by the action of TF pathway inhibitor (TFPI), which inactivates TF–VIIa and Xa by binding them in a quaternary complex.[10] The small amount of thrombin generated is able to activate the coagulation co-factors V and VIII and in the cell-based model of Hoffman, the subsequent steps take place on the phospholipid surface of activated platelets where factors Va and VIIIa are bound.[11] Factor VIIIa augments the activity of the previously activated IXa by five orders of magnitude and thus generates more Xa, which, with the now active Va, is able to generate substantial amounts of thrombin (Fig. 3.2). These feedback loops result in the rapid burst of thrombin, which is the hallmark of effective coagulation (Fig. 3.3). Although fibrin clot formation *in vitro* occurs early in this system and may even precede the thrombin burst, it is ineffective without the bulk thrombin generation that follows.[12] This may be because the rate of fibrin formation is important and/or because the additional thrombin is required for inhibition of fibrinolysis (see below). The importance of the phospholipid surface provided by activated platelets is illustrated by the bleeding defect in the (albeit rare) Scott syndrome in which this activity is absent.[13]

The role of factor XI in this system was for a long while ambiguous. It is now known that it too is activated by thrombin on phospholipid surfaces and can thus generate more IXa to further boost thrombin generation. This appears to be important in some circumstances when trauma is major or fibrinolysis very active.[14]

As the fibrin forms, thrombin also activates factor XIII, a process for which fibrin has co-factor activity.[15] Cross linking of the forming protofibrils and bundles forms a dense mesh of fibrin strands. More rapid thrombin formation results in a denser fibrin mesh, more resistant to fibrinolysis.[16]

After the clot: inhibition of coagulation

Thrombin is active in free solution so that the rapid generation of so much thrombin is potentially lethal, and is limited by an equally powerful and complex inhibitory system.[17,18] Thrombin diffusing away from the site of coagulation will be captured in two ways. Firstly, it will bind to thrombomodulin (TM) expressed on the surface of normal endothelium. In doing so the substrate specificity of thrombin changes so that its preferred substrate is now protein C, which it activates by specific proteolytic cleavage.[19] Activated protein C (APC) in concert with its co-factor protein S, then inactivates factors Va and (probably) VIIIa by further specific proteolytic cleavage thus shutting down coagulation. Secondly, thrombin is captured and neutralized by antithrombin facilitated by heparan molecules on the endothelial wall.[20] Antithrombin will also neutralize the serine proteases factors IXa and Xa. In this way, the clot formed is surrounded by an anticoagulant ring suppressing and limiting the spread of procoagulant activity.[21]

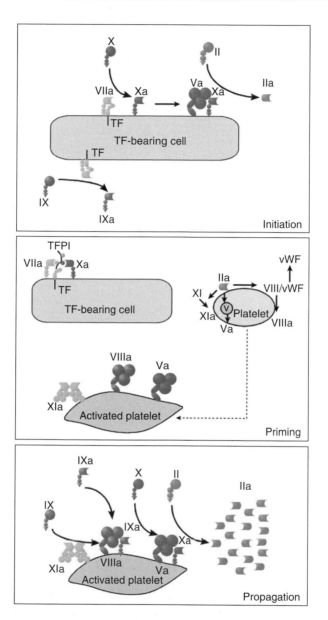

Figure 3.2 Cell-based model of coagulation. In this scheme, coagulation occurs in three phases: initiation, priming and propagation. In the initiation, factor VIIa bound to TF activates factor IX and also X. Factor Xa then activates factor V on the TF-bearing cell, complexes with factor Va, and converts a small amount of II to IIa. In the priming phase, the small amount of initial IIa activates platelets, causing release of granule contents including factor V, activates factors V, XI and VIII/by cleaving it from VWF/. Co-factors bind to the platelet surface before their respective enzymes. The factor VIIa–TF complex is shut down through the action of the TFPI in complex with factor Xa. In the propagation phase, factor IXa generated by factor VIIa–TF binds to the activated platelets and subsequently activates factor X. This factor IXa is supplemented by factor IXa generated on the platelet surface by factor XIa. Factor Xa then moves directly into a protected complex with factor Va, resulting in a burst of thrombin generation. Redrawn with permission from Monroe *et al.*[11]

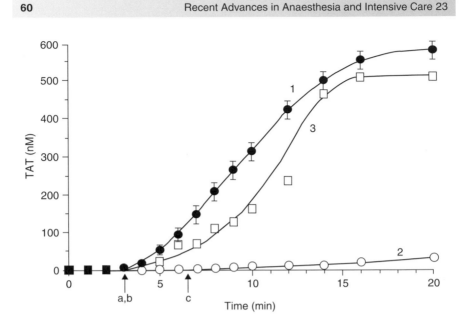

Figure 3.3 The influence of factor VIII on thrombin generation in whole blood. Thrombin generation (thrombin–antithrombin III complex, TAT) is initiated by 25 pM TF in normal (1) and haemophilia A blood without replacement (2) and with recombinant factor VIII (3). Arrows indicate clotting time in normal (a) and haemophilia A blood with (b) and without (c) replacement. Redrawn with permission from Butena and Mann. Biochemistry (Mosc) 2002; 67: 5–15.

Fibrinolysis

The fibrin clot is a temporary structure, achieving haemostasis pending the restoration of the normal vessel wall by healing. As fibrinogen is cleaved, binding sites on fibrin for tissue plasminogen activator (tPA) and plasminogen are exposed. Their consequent juxtaposition facilitates activation of plasminogen to plasmin which can then commence degradation of the clot.[22] Unopposed fibrinolysis can result in a bleeding disorder, but it too has inhibitory mechanisms to contend with: access to the fibrin strands is limited by factor XIII mediated cross linking and plasmin can be inactivated by antiplasmin, present both in plasma and bound to the fibrin. Finally, the lysine residues, to which tPA and plasminogen bind, are removed by the thrombin-activated fibrinolysis inhibitor (TAFI) which is also activated by TM-bound thrombin. It is this action of thrombin that seems to be most dependent on the additional enzyme generated by Factor XI activation.[23] The action of plasmin breaks fibrin down into numerous fragments, most of which could equally have been produced by the breakdown of fibrinogen; these are referred to as fibrin(ogen) degradation products (FDPs). However, some fragments, notably those between the D domains of adjacent fibrin molecules, consist of two fragments from cross-linked fibrin chains and are called D-dimers. D-dimers can only be

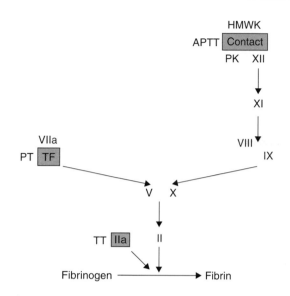

Figure 3.4 The pathways utilized by coagulation screening tests. The coagulation factor requirements of the basic coagulation screening tests are shown. The triggers are given in the shaded boxes. Thus the APTT is triggered by the provision of a contact-activating surface. Traditionally this was the surface of a glass tube but in modern analysers is celite, kaolin, elagic acid or micronized silica. The path to generation of a fibrin clot then requires factors XI, IX, VIII, X, V and II (prothrombin), prekallikrein and high-molecular-weight kininogen (HMWK). Similarly the PT is triggered by addition of TF (thromboplastin) and requires factors VII, X, V and II. The simplest test is the thrombin time (TT) in which added thrombin is used to clot fibrinogen. Thus, the TT needs only fibrinogen and the absence of thrombin inhibitors, mostly commonly heparin. The pattern of abnormalities allows the factor deficiency to be localized.

produced from the breakdown of fibrin and, therefore, indicate that the coagulation mechanism has been activated.[24]

Tests of coagulation

The tests of coagulation most frequently used in hospital practice are the prothrombin time (PT) and activated partial thromboplastin time (APTT). The pathways utilized by these tests are shown in Figure 3.4. It is an unfortunate accident of history that the laboratory tests of coagulation which we have developed, bear only a limited relationship to the events *in vivo* described above.[25] There are two important differences; firstly the contact activation system used to initiate the APTT does not have any role in normal coagulation *in vivo*. Thus, the very long APTT resulting from, for example, factor XII deficiency is not accompanied by any haemorrhagic tendency in the patient, whereas the prolonged APTT resulting from factor VIII deficiency clearly is. Secondly, the amount of TF present in the thromboplastins used for initiating the PT is so large that the function of TFPI is not seen and the test becomes independent of factors VIII,

Table 3.1 Haemorrhagic disorders not detected by screening tests (PT, APTT and TT)

- Mild factor deficiencies
- von Willebrand disease
- Factor XIII deficiency
- Platelet disorders
- Excessive fibrinolysis
- Vessel wall disorders
- Metabolic disorders (e.g. uraemia)

IX and XI. Therefore, although the trigger in the PT is the physiological one of TF, it does not detect the bleeding tendency associated with haemophilia (factor VIII or IX deficiency). Finally, because these tests are dependent on the levels of several different coagulation factors, and are subject to numerous confounding factors, their sensitivity is limited, so that mild but potentially significant factor deficiencies may not be detected. Nonetheless, once these shortcomings are understood, the tests can be usefully interpreted.[26]

A routine assessment of coagulation in hospital will usually comprise a platelet count, PT, APTT, fibrinogen and possibly a thrombin time (TT).[26] However, these reflect only a fraction of the mechanisms described above and, thus, a large number of haemorrhagic states remain routinely undetected (Table 3.1). The primary means of detecting or excluding a haemorrhagic state remains in the clinical history. They are of course also insensitive to prothrombotic states, but detection of these is rarely a matter of urgency. From a practical point of view, the most useful additional test is an assessment of primary haemostasis and the most widely used is now probably the platelet function analyser (PFA) 100 (Behring Dade)™.[27,28] This provides a sensitive assessment of primary haemostasis and a normal result depends on adequate VWF–platelet activity and a normal haematocrit. It is simple and quick to perform but requires purchase of a special device. Historically, the bleeding time has fulfilled this function, but it has poor sensitivity and reproducibility.

Hereditary Disorders of Haemostasis

Some hereditary disorders of the systems described above can result in extremely severe bleeding tendencies. However, these rarely pose a diagnostic problem as they are diagnosed in childhood and treatment programmes are established from an early age. Paradoxically, it is those individuals with mild and previously unsuspected bleeding disorders who are likely to cause most problems at times of surgery or trauma. In addition many individuals inhabit the large grey area between clearly normal and abnormal which poses difficult diagnostic problems.

Hereditary disorders of primary haemostasis

Clinical features

These arise from disorders of collagen, platelets or VWF and vary from the rare, and potentially life threatening such as Glanzmann's thrombasthenia, to common and frequently mild forms of von Willebrand disease.[29] Minor platelet function defects are also extremely common. They are all characterized by easy bruising, prolonged bleeding from superficial cuts and bleeding from mucosal surfaces such as epistaxes and menorrhagia. Trauma and surgery will of course produce bleeding which is immediate and prolonged. Inheritance is autosomal dominant or recessive (*cf.* haemophilia). The diagnosis of these mild disorders is fraught with the difficulty of establishing a normal range: there is a large grey area between the clearly abnormal and the clearly normal, and the occupants of this area are not always best served by being labelled as 'bleeders'.[30]

The problem is best illustrated by von Willebrand disease, where diagnosis is complicated by:[31]

- *The effect of ABO blood group*: Individuals with blood group O have VWF levels 25–30% lower than those with non-O groups. Consequently, a blood group O normal range has a much lower limit than a blood group A normal range (35.6 versus 48 iu/ml), and lower also than a normal range based on the general population.[32] Thus many people with blood group O have apparently subnormal VWF levels. Although this may explain the over-representation of blood group O individuals in groups of patients registered with von Willebrand disease, it is clear that most group O people do not bleed excessively and that a diagnosis of von Willebrand disease should not be made solely on the basis of slightly low VWF levels.

- *Variation over time*: VWF is an acute phase reactant and is easily elevated by stress, infection and exercise. Several estimations may be required to establish a representative value.

- *Incomplete penetrance making family histories unreliable.*

- *The poor predictive value of minor bleeding symptoms*: For example, in a study of children who did not bleed excessively after tonsillectomy (a fairly robust test of haemostatic ability) 36% had a history of easy bruising and 39% a history of epistaxes.[33]

From a practical point of view, the diagnosis has been aided considerably by the use of global screening devices such as the platelet function analyser, PFA100. This has the virtue of summating VWF and platelet functional activity to give an overall measure of primary haemostatic capacity. It is also sensitive to the platelet count and haematocrit.[34] The PFA100 has a very good sensitivity for von Willebrand disease and although there is no study correlating results directly with bleeding, repeatedly normal results make a significant disorder of primary haemostasis very unlikely.[28]

Treatment

Many mild forms of von Willebrand disease (Type 1) will respond to desmopressin (1-desamino-8-D-arginine vasopressin, DDAVP) by elevating their levels to normal haemostatic level.[35] Mild platelet disorders will also respond well, possibly due to a compensatory effect of increased amounts of high-molecular-weight VWF molecules and also some indirect platelet-activating effect. The defects in more severe platelet disorders such as Glanzmann's and von Willebrand disease Type 2 or 3 do not respond to DDAVP and appropriate replacement therapy is required; that is, platelets or an intermediate purity factor VIII concentrate containing adequate amounts of high-molecular-weight VWF multimers. In addition, DDAVP should not be given to patients under the age of 2 years (risk of hyponatremia and seizures) or with arterial disease or over 60 years of age (risk of myocardial infarction or stroke).[35] Recombinant VWF is not yet available. A single pool of platelets contains the platelets from six donors ($>240 \times 10^9$/l) and is sufficient to achieve haemostasis under normal circumstances. Platelets and cryoprecipitate are also useful sources of VWF in emergency or if concentrates are ineffective.

Hereditary disorders of coagulation

Clinical features

The archetypal disorder of coagulation is severe haemophilia arising from virtually complete deficiency of either factor VIII or IX. This is characterized by repeated and essentially spontaneous bleeding into deep structures such as joints and muscles. Clinically the two disorders (referred to as haemophilia A and B, respectively) are indistinguishable.[36] The superficial bleeding typical of von Willebrand disease such as nosebleeds is not seen in haemophilia and the bleeding time is normal due to normal platelet–VWF function. Even deeper cuts may appear to stop bleeding but the clot formed is friable and inadequate; it soon falls off and bleeding restarts. Thus bleeding in disorders of coagulation is characteristically delayed and a stop–start cycle may be repeated many times before the diagnosis is

Table 3.2 Severity of bleeding in haemophilia

Severity	Severe	Moderate	Mild
Factor VIII level (%)	<2	2–5	5–40
Bleeding pattern	Spontaneous Into muscles, joints and deep soft tissues	After minor trauma Bleeds into joints rare	Only bleed after surgery or major injury

made. The reasons for the initial cessation and then resumption of bleeding are complex. Partly it is attributable to the initial formation of a platelet plug, which disintegrates without a supporting fibrin mesh. Some fibrin is formed but the rate of thrombin production is slow resulting in only a loose meshwork and inadequate activation of TAFI so that the fibrin is more readily broken down by the fibrinolytic system. In the absence of adequate thrombin generation, bleeding is prolonged and historically patients would die over several weeks from slow but inexorable blood loss.

Diagnosis in severe cases is usually straightforward and made in infancy. However, patients with mild forms of haemophilia have relatively little trouble in day-to-day life and are frequently not diagnosed until they undergo surgery much later in life. In this way they are potentially more dangerous than the severe types (Table 3.2). Another potentially hazardous patient is the female heterozygous (carrier) of haemophilia. The assumption in families with haemophilia (and of many doctors) is that the men suffer from haemophilia and the women carry it but are unaffected. However, due to the effects of X chromosome inactivation, they frequently have levels of <30%, putting them at the same order of risk as men with mild haemophilia. During pregnancy, factor VIII (but not factor IX) levels rise naturally thus correcting the defect for most carriers and further disguising the problem.[37]

Once bleeding has started in a haemophiliac it will rarely stop in any satisfactory time or fashion without replacement therapy (or DDAVP for mild factor VIII deficiency). It is important not to be misled by the apparent cessation described above.

Factor VIII and IX deficiencies are prominent because they are both sex linked, and thus readily apparent in male hemizygotes. Other coagulation factor deficiencies are autosomal recessive and thus not so frequently encountered except in communities where intermarriage is more common. They each have their particular features and different levels are required for normal haemostasis.[38]

Disorders of fibrinolysis

Hereditary disorders of fibrinolysis are rare and frequently less severe than might be expected. Plasminogen activation inhibitor-1 (PAI-1) deficiency is described in a small number of patients and results in a mild bleeding tendency similar to that seen in mild forms of haemophilia.[39] A similar effect is seen in antiplasmin deficiency which in some cases has been more severe. However, plasminogen deficiency itself appears to be surprisingly mild and has a dubious association with thrombosis.[40,41]

Thrombotic disorders

Although something of an oversimplification, it is useful to think of the coagulation system as representing a balance between procoagulant and anticoagulant forces, disturbance of which may lead to haemorrhage or thrombosis. Thus deficiency of function on the part of the anticoagulant factors results in an increased tendency to thrombosis. The classic thrombophilic traits arise from deficiency of antithrombin protein C or protein S. They remain the most powerful genetic traits (relative risks of thrombosis shown in Table 3.3) but are rare and relatively infrequent explanations for thrombosis. More recently it has been recognized that excess of procoagulant factors also has a similar effect, in keeping with the balance analogy. Thus high levels of factor VIII, prothrombin, factors IX and XI,

Table 3.3 Prothrombotic traits and their associated risk of a first thrombotic event

State	Frequency in patients with first episode thrombosis (%)	OR for thrombosis (95% CI)
Anticoagulant deficiency		
Antithrombin	1–2	25–50
Protein C	2–4	10–20
Protein S	2–4	10–20
Procoagulant excess		
Factor V Leiden	20	6.6 (3.6–12.0)
Factor VIII (>1.5)	24	4.8 (2.3–10)
Prothrombin	6	2.8 (1.4–5.6)
Factor XI (>1.21)	20	2.2 (1.5–3.2)
Factor IX (>1.29)	20	2.5 (1.6–3.9)
Fibrinolysis		
TAFI	14	1.7 (1.1–2.5)
Factor XIII (Val34)	63	1.8 (1.2–2.6)
Dysfibrinogenemia	1	

CI: confidence interval; OR: odds ratio.

and fibrinogen itself have all been shown to increase the risk of thrombosis.[42] However, only for prothrombin and to a limited extent for fibrinogen, is the genetic basis understood. Even when a powerful thrombotic trait such as antithrombin deficiency is present, thrombosis is not inevitable. This is in keeping with the multifactorial model of thrombosis in which multiple factors, congenital and acquired, including most importantly age, combine to lift the tendency to thrombosis above a threshold level so that abnormal or inappropriate coagulation takes place. Typical acquired factors include surgery, malignancy, immobility, pregnancy and the combined oral contraceptive pill but in some cases, such as fractured neck of femur, the acquired stimulus is so powerful that virtually all patients form a thrombus irrespective of their prior risk.

The best known of thrombophilic traits is factor V Leiden. This variant of procoagulant factor V reaches polymorphic frequency in the white European population and its distribution extends around the southern coast of the Mediterranean through the Middle East and into northern India. The mutation abolishes the protein C cleavage site in factor V and thus delays factor V inactivation. Although present at frequencies of 3–10% in Europe, the effect is relatively mild: the risk of thrombosis is increased approximately 5-fold and only 30–40% of heterozygotes will have a thrombosis by the age of 60 years. Homozygotes are more severely affected and have a relative risk estimated at 80-fold.

Acquired Disorders of Coagulation

Intractable haemorrhage in hospital practice

As discussed above, it is quite possible for the milder forms of inherited disorders of coagulation or platelet function to present late in life after a surgical procedure and this possibility should be borne in mind when dealing with unexpectedly prolonged bleeding. It is also true that such bleeding often has a structural basis rather than reflecting a defect in the haemostatic mechanism: this might be surgical, unrecognized trauma or some kind of vascular abnormality. Post-partum haemorrhage may fall at least partly into this group. However, intractable haemorrhage in hospital practice usually represents an acquired disorder of haemostasis (Table 3.4). If an appropriate history is obtained then it is often possible to distinguish between acquired and congenital bleeding disorders but there may be no time for this in the acute situation.

Management of intractable haemorrhage is therefore a matter of judgement based on limited data. Some particular examples and their management

---

Table 3.4 Acquired disorders of haemostasis

- Dilutional coagulopathy
- DIC
- Liver failure
- Vitamin K deficiency
- An acquired coagulation factor inhibitor (antibody)
- Cardiopulmonary bypass
- Drug induced (including anticoagulants)
- Uraemia
- Thrombocytopaenia*

---

* Thrombocytopaenia is included for completenesss but has its own differential diagnosis and should be considered separately from the others here.

---

are discussed below. The mainstay of management is of course diagnosis. However, in the emergency situation this counsel of perfection is often not practicable. Rapid and adequate replacement therapy appropriate to the situation is crucial and should not be withheld pending the results of investigations. It is nonetheless important to obtain plasma samples prior to replacement, which can be analysed as treatment progresses or at a later date.

Dilutional coagulopathy

The most common reason for prolonged bleeding and deranged coagulation in hospital practice is dilutional coagulopathy, largely the result of inadequate plasma replacement. Standard resuscitation protocols will replace red blood cells (RBCs) as needed to maintain oxygen delivery. In many cases by the time it is clearly an emergency, the blood loss would have exceeded blood volume and dilutional anticoagulation would have taken place. Many protocols for replacement therapy have not been updated to take account of the fact that virtually all plasma is now removed from red cell units.[43]

Previous studies report that the risk of bleeding is increased when the PT ratio is >1.5 and the fibrinogen <0.8 g/l.[43,44] Computer modelling of an acutely exsanguinating patient shows that to prevent dilutional coagulopathy (as indicated by PT ratio >1.5), a fresh-frozen plasma (FFP): packed RBC (PRBC) ratio of 2:3 should be used. Data indicate that the PT is the most sensitive parameter of dilutional coagulopathy and so fibrinogen and the APTT are, thus, also kept in the haemostatic range. Moreover, the model shows that FFP replacement should be begun before 3 units of RBC are given. Where massive blood loss is anticipated, from the nature of the trauma, the procedure or the clinical situation, then plasma replacement should begin as soon as possible. The corresponding ratio for platelets is 8:10 or approximately one platelet pool for 8 units RBC.[44]

Disseminated intravascular coagulation

Disseminated intravascular coagulation (DIC) most frequently arises from a breakdown in the separation of intravascular coagulation factors from their extravascular triggers.[45] In brief, this amounts to intravascular exposure of TF, which is certainly the mechanism in sepsis, trauma and malignancy. TF is exposed on the malignant or damaged cells or presented on the surface of monocytes in response to lipopolysaccharide (LPS) or interleukin-6 (IL-6). These factors may stimulate the contact activation system too, but the consequence of this is largely bradykinin production and coagulation is driven by the normal TF pathway. Inhibition of the TF–VIIa pathway can block coagulation activation induced by sepsis in animal models.[46,47] The process is exacerbated by activation of endothelium by cytokines, especially TNFα. This causes downregulation of TM and possibly expression of TF which will have a procoagulant effect. High levels of PAI-1 from activated endothelium probably facilitate deposition of fibrin and consequent organ dysfunction. High levels of PAI-1 have been shown to be a predictor of poor outcome in meningococcal sepsis.[48] The result is widespread activation of coagulation with consumption and depletion of clotting factors resulting on the one hand in a bleeding tendency but on the other in intravascular deposition of fibrin and organ dysfunction.

The diagnosis of DIC is usually straightforward when prolongation of clotting tests and thrombocytopaenia are present in the appropriate clinical context. It may be confused, and indeed may coexist, with dilutional coagulopathy. Useful distinguishing features are that thrombocytopaenia is early in DIC but late in dilution and hypofibrinogenemia is a late event in DIC.

Management of DIC relies on the treatment and reversal of the underlying cause. If bleeding is present then aggressive replacement therapy with plasma and platelets is required. Cryoprecipitate is useful if the fibrinogen is particularly low. Until recently the beneficial effects of interventions based on the coagulation system that were seen in animal models could not be reproduced in clinical studies. However, one recent and much analysed study showed a benefit from treatment with APC.[49]

The role of heparin, which was not randomized in this trial, has not been clarified. Nor has the question as to whether the protein C needs to be activated; for example, there is considerable experience of using protein C with significant benefit in meningococcal septicaemia.[50]

Drugs and anticoagulants

Most hospital doctors are familiar with the anticoagulant effects of unfractionated heparin and even when there is doubt about its administration, the characteristic pattern of grossly prolonged TT, prolonged APTT and relatively unaffected PT is easily recognized. It is important to note that the newer low-molecular-weight heparins (LMWHs) may be present in therapeutic amounts without any abnormality of these tests being apparent. Detection and assay therefore requires a specific anti-factor Xa activity assay. Most doctors will also have some familiarity with using protamine to reverse the effect of heparin. There is an unfounded assumption that this will not work for LMWH but in fact approximately 50%, and in some cases more, of the activity is reversible in this way.[51]

In contrast there is considerable ignorance about warfarin reversal despite the publication of comprehensive guidelines. While vitamin K is surprisingly quick in restoring coagulation factor levels after 6–12 h, immediate reversal requires replacement therapy. FFP is very slow and ineffective at achieving this, and the method of choice is prothrombin complex concentrates, which contain factors X, IX, II and often (preferably) VII, and protein C: complete reversal of warfarin effect can be achieved in a matter of minutes.[52,53]

Factor deficiencies

Routine coagulation tests may point to a specific factor deficiency if one is disproportionately prolonged. As pointed out above, this may represent the late presentation of a (usually mild) congenital coagulation disorder, however, acquired disorders are also encountered, most commonly of anti-factor VIII antibodies (acquired haemophilia). These are most common in the elderly and mostly idiopathic although some are associated with other autoimmune disorders and some follow pregnancy.[54] Acquired hypoprothrombinaemia is encountered as a rare complication of lupus erythematosus and acquired von Willebrand syndrome may arise in association with paraproteinaemia or myeloproliferative disorders.[55] These problems are among the most difficult of coagulation disorders to manage and haematological advice should be sought.

Management of Bleeding Disorders

In generalized disorders of coagulation, such as DIC and dilutional coagulopathy, plasma and platelets are appropriate replacement therapy. RBCs will be needed to maintain the circulation but do not now supply any coagulation factors. Hence as noted above, in the face of uncontrolled haemorrhage plasma replacement should be proportional to the RBC and begun early. In some circumstances, usually when an element of DIC is present, the fibrinogen may be particularly low, in which case cryoprecipitate is useful.[56]

Cryoprecipitate also contains significant amounts of VWF, and factors VIII and XIII. A dose of 10 units can be given if the fibrinogen is <0.8 g/l.

When a specific factor deficiency is identified, then in most cases concentrates are available, which due to their small volume and high concentration are much more efficient at restoring haemostasis. Indeed the only coagulation factor for which a concentrate is not available is factor V.

Useful adjunctive non-plasma agents include DDAVP, which is useful for suspected von Willebrand disease, minor platelet disorders, mild haemophilia and uraemia. Its principal effect is to release endothelial stores of VWF, but it should be avoided in the young (hyponatremia) or the elderly (risk of vascular occlusion).[57]

Recombinant factor VIIa

Not infrequently patients continue to bleed despite all the efforts outlined above. The surgeon may have taken the patient back to theatre and been unable to identify a responsible bleeding point, plasma replacement therapy has been aggressive and the coagulation screen now has results with which haemostasis might reasonably be expected and normal functional platelets have been given. In these circumstances there has been much interest in using recombinant factor VIIa (factor VIIa), an agent originally developed for use in haemophiliacs with anti-factor VIII antibodies. It appears to work by directly activating Factor X on the surface of platelets in the absence of TF for which very high concentrations are required. Randomized, controlled clinical trials, evaluating the use of recombinant factor VIIa in trauma and patients undergoing certain surgical procedures, are either in development or ongoing, but are unlikely to address the problem of refractory haemorrhage in general.[58] A recent trial showed evidence of benefit in prostate surgery[59] and there is a reasonable amount of anecdotal experience.[60]

Tranexomic acid

Tranexamic acid is widely used as an adjunctive haemostatic agent when treating haemophilia. It acts by binding to blocking binding of plasminogen and tPA to fibrin and is particularly useful in situations where fibrinolytic activity is high such as the oropharynx. Its use should be avoided where the deposition of insoluble fibrin may be harmful such as haematuria and in Disseminated Intravascular Coagulation. Its utility in haemophilia seems to arise from the failure to activate TAFI when thrombin generation is suboptimal.

Trasylol

Trasylol has found a role in some forms of surgery such as cardiopulmonary bypass but its mode of action is still not clear. Originally thought to reduce blood loss by inhibiting fibrinolysis, there is now evidence that it may help by preserving platelet function.[61] Fibrin glue, usually a combination of fibrin and thrombin, can be used topically for areas of diffusely haemorrhagic or oozing surgical fields. There is no evidence that these latter two agents have any role outside of surgical bleeding.

Summary

Normal haemostasis is achieved by a complex mechanism comprising a balance between pro- and anti-coagulant forces. hereditary or acquired deficiency of factors on either side of this balance may result in a pro-thrombotic or a haemorrhagic tendency. The system is continually active at a low rate which allows it to be rapidly responsive to haemorrhagic challenge. Separation of the physiological trigger for coagulation (TF) from the effector enzymes in plasma is essential for controlling this system. Improved understanding allows us effectively to manipulate this system and treat these disorders for therapeutic benefit.

References

1. Kulkarni S, Dopheide SM, Yap CL et al. A revised model of platelet aggregation. J Clin Invest 2000; 105: 783–791.
2. Ruggeri ZM. Old concepts and new developments in the study of platelet aggregation. J Clin Invest 2000; 105: 699–701.
3. Goto S, Ikeda Y, Saldivar E, Ruggeri ZM. Distinct mechanisms of platelet aggregation as a consequence of different shearing flow conditions. J Clin Invest 1998; 101: 479–486.
4. Brass LF. Thrombin and platelet activation. Chest 2003; 124: 18S–25S.
5. Nieswandt B, Watson SP. Platelet–collagen interaction: is GPVI the central receptor? Blood 2003; 102: 449–461.
6. Ni H, Yuen PS, Papalia JM et al. Plasma fibronectin promotes thrombus growth and stability in injured arterioles. Proc Natl Acad Sci USA 2003; 100: 2415–2419.
7. McVey JH. Tissue factor pathway. Best Pract Res Clin Haematol 1999; 12: 361–372.
8. Morrissey JH. Tissue factor: an enzyme cofactor and a true receptor. Thromb Haemost 2001; 86: 66–74.
9. Butenas S, Mann KG. Blood coagulation. Biochemistry (Mosc) 2002; 67: 3–12.
10. Kato H. Regulation of functions of vascular wall cells by tissue factor pathway inhibitor: basic and clinical aspects. Arterioscler Thromb Vasc Biol 2002; 22: 539–548.
11. Monroe DM, Hoffman M, Roberts HR. Platelets and thrombin generation. Arterioscler Thromb Vasc Biol 2002; 22: 1381–1389.

12. Cawthern KM, van't Veer C, Lock JB, DiLorenzo ME, Branda RF, Mann KG. Blood coagulation in hemophilia A and hemophilia C. Blood 1998; 91: 4581–4592.

13. Solum NO. Procoagulant expression in platelets and defects leading to clinical disorders. Arterioscler Thromb Vasc Biol 1999; 19: 2841–2846.

14. Broze Jr GJ, Gailani D. The role of factor XI in coagulation. Thromb Haemost 1993; 70: 72–74.

15. Philippou H, Rance J, Myles T et al. Roles of low specificity and cofactor interaction sites on thrombin during factor XIII activation. Competition for cofactor sites on thrombin determines its fate. J Biol Chem 2003; 278: 32020–32026.

16. Wolberg AS, Monroe DM, Roberts HR, Hoffman M. Elevated prothrombin results in clots with an altered fiber structure: a possible mechanism of the increased thrombotic risk. Blood 2003; 101: 3008–3013.

17. Lane DA, Mannucci PM, Bauer KA et al. Inherited thrombophilia: Part 2 [erratum appears in Thromb Haemost 1997 May; 77(5): 1047]. Thromb Haemost 1996; 76: 824–834.

18. Lane DA, Mannucci PM, Bauer KA et al. Inherited thrombophilia: Part 1. Thromb Haemost 1996; 76: 651–662.

19. Esmon CT. The protein C pathway. Chest 2003; 124: 26S–32S.

20. van Boven HH, Lane DA. Antithrombin and its inherited deficiency states. Semin Hematol 1997; 34: 188–204.

21. Roemisch J, Gray E, Hoffmann JN, Wiedermann CJ. Antithrombin: a new look at the actions of a serine protease inhibitor. Blood Coagul Fibrin 2002; 13: 657–670.

22. Medved L, Nieuwenhuizen W. Molecular mechanisms of initiation of fibrinolysis by fibrin. Thromb Haemost 2003; 89: 409–419.

23. Bouma BN, Meijers JC. Thrombin-activatable fibrinolysis inhibitor (TAFI, plasma procarboxypeptidase B, procarboxypeptidase R, procarboxypeptidase U). J Thromb Haemost 2003; 1: 1566–1574.

24. Doolittle RF. X-ray crystallographic studies on fibrinogen and fibrin. J Thromb Haemost 2003; 1: 1559–1565.

25. Butenas S, van't Veer C, Cawthern K, Brummel KE, Mann KG. Models of blood coagulation. Blood Coagul Fibrin 2000; 11: S9–S13.

26. Laffan M, Manning R. Investigation of haemostasis and bleeding tendency. In: Lewis SM, Bain B (eds) Practical Haematology, 9th ed. Edinburgh: Churchill Livingstone, 2000.

27. Nitu-Whalley IC, Lee CA, Brown SA, Riddell A, Hermans C. The role of the platelet function analyser (PFA-100) in the characterization of patients with von Willebrand's disease and its relationships with von Willebrand factor and the ABO blood group. Haemophilia 2003; 9: 298–302.

28. Fressinaud E, Veyradier A, Truchaud F et al. Screening for von Willebrand disease with a new analyzer using high shear stress: a study of 60 cases. Blood 1998; 91: 1325–1331.

29. Sadler JE, Mannucci PM, Berntorp E et al. Impact, diagnosis and treatment of von Willebrand disease. Thromb Haemost 2000; 84: 160–174.

30. Sadler JE. Von Willebrand disease type 1: a diagnosis in search of a disease. Blood 2003; 101: 2089–2093.

31. Laffan MA, Brown SA, Collins P et al. The diagnosis of von Willebrand disease: a guideline from the UK Haemophilia Centre Doctors' Organisation. Haemophilia 2004; 10: 199–217.

32. Gill JC, Endres-Brooks J, Bauer PJ, Marks Jr WJ, Montgomery RR. The effect of ABO blood group on the diagnosis of von Willebrand disease. Blood 1987; 69: 1691–1695.

33. Nosek-Cenkowska B, Cheang MS, Pizzi NJ, Israels ED, Gerrard JM. Bleeding/bruising symptomatology in children with and without bleeding disorders. Thromb Haemost 1991; 65: 237–241.

34. Harrison P, Robinson MS, Mackie IJ et al. Performance of the platelet function analyser PFA-100 in testing abnormalities of primary haemostasis. Blood Coagul Fibrin 1999; 10: 25–31.

35. Pasi KJ, Collins PW, Keeling D et al. Management of von Willebrand Disease: A guideline from the UK Haemophilia Centre Doctors' Organisation. Haemophilia 2004; 10: 218–231.

36. Mannucci PM, Tuddenham EG. The hemophilias – from royal genes to gene therapy [erratum appears in New Engl J Med 2001 Aug 2; 345(5): 384]. New Engl J Med 2001; 344: 1773–1779.

37. Clark P, Brennand J, Conkie JA, McCall F, Greer IA, Walker ID. Activated protein C sensitivity, protein C, protein S and coagulation in normal pregnancy. Thromb Haemost 1998; 79: 1166–1170.

38. Peyvandi F, Duga S, Akhavan S, Mannucci PM. Rare coagulation deficiencies. Haemophilia 2002; 8: 308–321.

39. Fay WP, Parker AC, Condrey LR, Shapiro AD. Human plasminogen activator inhibitor-1 (PAI-1) deficiency: characterization of a large kindred with a null mutation in the PAI-1 gene. Blood 1997; 90: 204–208.

40. Brandt JT. Plasminogen and tissue-type plasminogen activator deficiency as risk factors for thromboembolic disease. Arch Pathol Lab Med 2002; 126: 1376–1381.

41. Okamoto A, Sakata T, Mannami T et al. Population-based distribution of plasminogen activity and estimated prevalence and relevance to thrombotic diseases of plasminogen deficiency in the Japanese: the Suita Study. J Thromb Haemost 2003; 1: 2397–2403.

42. Greaves M. Thrombophilia. Clin Med 2001; 1: 432–435.

43. Anonymous. Guidelines for transfusion for massive blood loss. A publication of the British Society for Haematology. British Committee for Standardization in Haematology Blood Transfusion Task Force. Clin Lab Haematol 1988; 10: 265–273.

44. Hirshberg A, Dugas M, Banez EI, Scott BG, Wall Jr MJ, Mattox KL. Minimizing dilutional coagulopathy in exsanguinating hemorrhage: a computer simulation. J Trauma 2003; 54: 454–463.

45. Levi M. Current understanding of disseminated intravascular coagulation. Br J Haematol 2004; 124: 567–576.

46. de Jonge E, Dekkers PE, Creasey AA et al. Tissue factor pathway inhibitor dose-dependently inhibits coagulation activation without influencing the fibrinolytic and cytokine response during human endotoxemia. Blood 2000; 95: 1124–1129.

47. Levi M, ten Cate H, Bauer KA et al. Inhibition of endotoxin-induced activation of coagulation and fibrinolysis by pentoxifylline or by a monoclonal anti-tissue factor antibody in chimpanzees. J Clin Invest 1994; 93: 114–120.

48. Hermans PW, Hibberd ML, Booy R et al. 4G/5G promoter polymorphism in the plasminogen-activator-inhibitor-1 gene and outcome of meningococcal disease. Meningococcal Research Group. Lancet 1999; 354: 556–560.

49. Bernard GR, Vincent JL, Laterre PF et al. Efficacy and safety of recombinant human activated protein C for severe sepsis. New Engl J Med 2001; 344: 699–709.

50. White B, Livingstone W, Murphy C, Hodgson A, Rafferty M, Smith OP. An open-label study of the role of adjuvant hemostatic support with protein C replacement therapy in purpura fulminans-associated meningococcemia. Blood 2000; 96: 3719–3724.
51. Crowther MA, Berry LR, Monagle PT, Chan AK. Mechanisms responsible for the failure of protamine to inactivate low-molecular-weight heparin. Br J Haematol 2002; 116: 178–186.
52. Watson HG, Baglin T, Laidlaw SL, Makris M, Preston FE. A comparison of the efficacy and rate of response to oral and intravenous vitamin K in reversal of over-anticoagulation with warfarin. Br J Haematol 2001; 115: 145–149.
53. Makris M, Watson HG. The management of coumarin-induced over-anticoagulation annotation. Br J Haematol 2001; 114: 271–280.
54. Collins P, Macartney N, Davies R, Lees S, Giddings J, Majer R. A population based, unselected, consecutive cohort of patients with acquired haemophilia A. Br J Haematol 2004; 124: 86–90.
55. Federici AB, Rand JH, Bucciarelli P et al. Acquired von Willebrand syndrome: data from an international registry [erratum appears in Thromb Haemost 2000 Oct; 84(4): 739]. Thromb Haemost 2000; 84: 345–349.
56. Colvin BT. Management of disseminated intravascular coagulation. Br J Haematol 1998; 101: 15–17.
57. Mannucci PM. Desmopressin (DDAVP) in the treatment of bleeding disorders: the first 20 years. Blood 1997; 90: 2515–2521.
58. Martinowitz U, Kenet G, Segal E et al. Recombinant activated factor VII for adjunctive hemorrhage control in trauma. J Trauma 2001; 51: 431–438; discussion 438–439.
59. Friederich PW, Henny CP, Messelink EJ et al. Effect of recombinant activated factor VII on perioperative blood loss in patients undergoing retropubic prostatectomy: a double-blind placebo-controlled randomised trial [erratum appears in Lancet 2003 Mar 29; 361(9363): 1138]. Lancet 2003; 361: 201–205.
60. O'Connell NM, Perry DJ, Hodgson AJ, O'Shaughnessy DF, Laffan MA, Smith OP. Recombinant FV IIa in the management of uncontrolled hemorrhage. Transfusion 2003; 43: 1711–1716.
61. Poulis M, Manning R, Laffan M, Haskard DO, Taylor KM and Landis RC. "The antithrombotic effect of aprotinin: action mediated via the protease activated receptor 1." J Thorac Cardiovasc Surg 120 (2000) 370–378.

W. Schlack   D. Ebel

Anaesthetic agents and myocardial protection

Ischaemia–reperfusion of the heart commonly occurs in a variety of clinical situations such as during heart transplantation, coronary artery bypass grafting and valvular surgery. The anaesthctist may also encounter ischaemia–reperfusion injury without any surgical intervention, for example after transient myocardial ischaemia during anaesthetic induction. Depending on the severity and duration of ischaemia, lack of oxygen supply may result in reversible or irreversible damage to the myocardium. Early restoration of arterial blood flow combined with surgical measures to improve the ischaemic tolerance of the tissue, such as organ cooling or cardioplegic solutions, are the main therapeutic options currently used.

In recent years, new insights into the pathophysiological mechanisms involved have been gained, and it has also become clear that anaesthetic drugs can interfere with those mechanisms, providing either protection or being inert, or even increasing the damage by blocking protective mechanisms. Thus, anaesthetic drugs may interfere substantially with the process of perioperative myocardial protection – a new concept still often ignored by both surgeons and anaesthetists.

If an ischaemia–reperfusion situation should occur, there are three occasions when drugs may potentially interact with the injury process: during ischaemia, before ischaemia and after ischaemia (i.e. during reperfusion).

Interaction with Ischaemic Injury

The beneficial effect of volatile anaesthetics during myocardial ischaemia was observed in 1969 by Spieckermann and colleagues,[1] who found a prolongation of tolerance to global ischaemia and enhanced preservation of high energy compounds in dog hearts during halothane anaesthesia. Several studies demonstrated that volatile anaesthetics reduced myocardial oxygen demand during ischaemia, thereby reducing ischaemic damage.[2–4] In patients with coronary artery disease, isoflurane improved the tolerance to pacing-induced myocardial ischaemia.[5] Sevoflurane and desflurane also showed anti-ischaemic properties.[6–8] The mechanisms behind this protection may be the negative inotropic and negative chronotropic action of these volatile anaesthetic agents. In addition, volatile anaesthetics maintain myocardial energy stores and might increase collateral blood flow to the ischaemic area, thereby reducing the severity of ischaemia. However, the overall direct anti-ischaemic effect of these anaesthetic agents is relatively small when compared with their pre-ischaemic ('preconditioning') effect or their effects on reperfusion injury. Therefore, the clinical benefit from the direct anti-ischaemic action of these anaesthetics appears to be limited.

Effects against Reperfusion Injury

Definition

The term 'reperfusion injury' was defined as *'metabolic, functional and structural changes after restoration of coronary perfusion, which can be reduced or prohibited by modification of the reperfusion conditions'*.[9] Reperfusion injury can be divided into non-lethal (reversible cellular damage) and lethal (irreversible damage).

Mechanisms and clinical manifestation of reperfusion injury

Non-lethal reperfusion injury includes myocardial dysrhythmias and post-ischaemic reduction of myocardial function. The reversible, but delayed recovery of myocardial function after complete restoration of coronary blood flow is called 'myocardial stunning',[10] The commonest clinical scenario is that of the patient who requires short-term inotropic support after discontinuation of cardiopulmonary bypass but who then makes a full recovery. Lethal reperfusion injury is characterized by irreversible cell death (myocardial necrosis) and can be divided into early phase (immediately at the beginning of reperfusion) and late phase myocardial damage (Fig. 4.1). The different characteristics of the reperfusion injury are caused

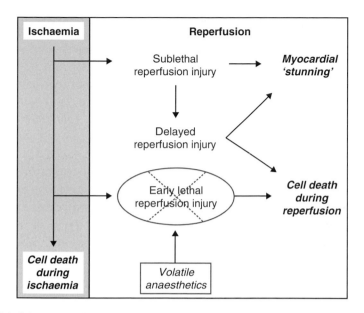

Figure 4.1 If the myocardium becomes ischaemic, it will die if the oxygen supply is not restored. However, reperfusion itself may lead to additional injury: reperfusion injury. If reperfusion occurs early, the myocardium survives and is only functionally impaired ('stunning'). Late reperfusion will result in cell death by reperfusion injury. Volatile anaesthetic agents can interact specifically with the pathophysiological mechanisms of lethal reperfusion injury and thereby reduce the amount of myocardial necrosis.

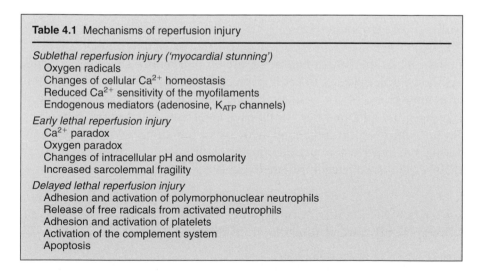

Table 4.1 Mechanisms of reperfusion injury

Sublethal reperfusion injury ('myocardial stunning')
  Oxygen radicals
  Changes of cellular Ca^{2+} homeostasis
  Reduced Ca^{2+} sensitivity of the myofilaments
  Endogenous mediators (adenosine, K_{ATP} channels)

Early lethal reperfusion injury
  Ca^{2+} paradox
  Oxygen paradox
  Changes of intracellular pH and osmolarity
  Increased sarcolemmal fragility

Delayed lethal reperfusion injury
  Adhesion and activation of polymorphonuclear neutrophils
  Release of free radicals from activated neutrophils
  Adhesion and activation of platelets
  Activation of the complement system
  Apoptosis

by distinct pathophysiological mechanisms (Table 4.1), which can be modified by therapeutic interventions. A recent review describes in more detail the pathophysiological mechanisms and how anaesthetic drugs can interact.[11]

Interaction of anaesthetics with reperfusion injury

In 1996, specific protection against myocardial reperfusion injury by halothane was described.[12] While all previous studies could not discriminate between anti-ischaemic effects and effects against reperfusion injury, this study demonstrated for the first time that modification of the reperfusion conditions by administration of a common volatile anaesthetic specifically reduced reperfusion damage. A similar cardioprotective effect was confirmed for enflurane, isoflurane, sevoflurane and desflurane and the noble gas xenon under a variety of experimental conditions *in vitro* and *in vivo*; cardioprotection against reperfusion damage was also maintained when the heart was already protected against ischaemic damage by cardioplegic solutions.[11] The amount of cardioprotection in all these studies was substantial, leading to an infarction size reduction of about 50%. Several specific mechanisms could be identified: a direct action on the myocardial cell limiting immediate damage by an interaction with the ryanodine receptor of the sarcoplasmic reticulum[13] and an action against neutrophile-mediated secondary damage[14] (Fig. 4.1). While there is a large body of laboratory evidence for a specific cardioprotective effect of the inhalational anaesthetics against reperfusion injury, only one clinical study has confirmed these findings. In patients undergoing coronary artery bypass grafting, 1.7 vol. % of isoflurane given for the first 15 min after the release of the aortic cross-clamp led to a substantial reduction in the need for inotropic support and to a reduction in myocardial damage assessed by postoperative troponin release.[15]

Unlike inhalational anaesthetics, the use of intravenous anaesthetic agents has shown little evidence of cardioprotection during ischaemia–reperfusion situations. Propofol, for example, was known to be an oxygen free-radical scavenger and inhibited Ca^{2+} influx across plasma membranes, but its use did not improve post-ischaemic myocardial function.[16] When given only during the reperfusion period, propofol provided no protective effect against cellular damage in isolated rat hearts.[17]

Effects of Anaesthetics Before Ischaemia: Preconditioning

The concept of preconditioning

It would appear that most cells have an endogenous protection system that, if activated before ischaemia, partially protects the cells against the consequences of ischaemia–reperfusion. The protection mechanism is called 'preconditioning', and the activating stimulus can be a short period of ischaemia, oxidative stress, a small change in temperature or some drugs.

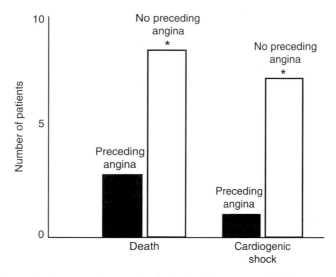

Figure 4.2 Patients with preceding angina (filled bars) have a much better outcome after myocardial infarction compared with patients without preinfarction angina (open bars) * = $P < 0.05$. Assuming that angina may be the physiological equivalent to ischaemic preconditioning, this finding would underline the clinical importance of the preconditioning mechanism. Modified from Ref. [21].

Preconditioning was first discovered in the myocardium by Murry and co-workers[18] when they tried to increase infarction size in dogs by multiple periods of short ischaemia preceding a longer period of ischaemia. Surprisingly, infarction size was not increased but reduced by more than 50%, if the infarction-inducing long ischaemic period was preceded by short ischaemic periods. A number of studies have confirmed these findings in all species tested and also in different tissues. The first, early phase of protection ('classic or early preconditioning', EPC) begins shortly after the preconditioning stimulus and disappears after 2–3 h. Cardioprotection from preconditioning reappears 12–24 h after the initial preconditioning stimulus, and lasts for 2–3 days. This phenomenon has been termed 'late preconditioning' (LPC) or the 'second window of protection'.[19] Mechanisms of ischaemic preconditioning have been reviewed.[20]

If one assumes that for the heart, angina is the physiological equivalent of preconditioning, the findings of Kloner and colleagues[21] underline the clinical importance of this phenomenon: patients in whom a myocardial infarction is preceded by angina have a much better outcome in terms of survival (Fig. 4.2). During cardiac surgery, mechanical ischaemic preconditioning of the heart can be employed as an effective adjunct to myocardial protection. However, it requires repeated aortic cross-clamping for the on-pump procedures and therefore may not attain widespread use.[22] Pharmacological preconditioning may be more useful, as some anaesthetic agents can stimulate preconditioning while others may block it.

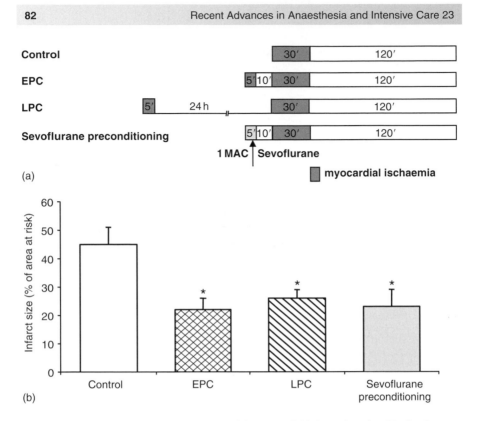

(a)

(b)

Figure 4.3 (a) Experimental programme and (b) myocardial infarct size after 30 min of regional myocardial ischaemia followed by 120 min of reperfusion * = $P < 0.05$ versus Control. Five minutes inhalation of one minimal alveolar concentration (MAC) sevoflurane has a similar infarct size reducing effect as the 'endogenous' cardioprotective mechanisms 'EPC' and 'LPC'. Values: time in minutes. Modified from Ref. [24].

Pharmacological preconditioning with anaesthetic agents

Not only myocardial ischaemia, but also pharmacological stimulation by volatile anaesthetic agents can elicit this cardioprotective effect. Figure 4.3 gives an example of the extent of infarction size reduction seen after only short administration of a volatile anaesthetic.[23]

Interestingly, the inert gas xenon is similar to the volatile anaesthetics, inducing a profound preconditioning effect despite being haemodynamically 'inert'.[24] Anaesthetic-induced preconditioning not only reduces infarction size, but also post-ischaemic myocardial contractile dysfunction ('myocardial stunning') and endothelial dysfunction in various experimental models. To induce these changes that persist long after the volatile anaesthetic has been discontinued, the anaesthetic must have lasting effects on intracellular protein and signal transduction. A detailed discussion of the molecular mechanisms is beyond the scope of this chapter, but the interested reader is referred to two excellent recent reviews.[25,26] Figure 4.4

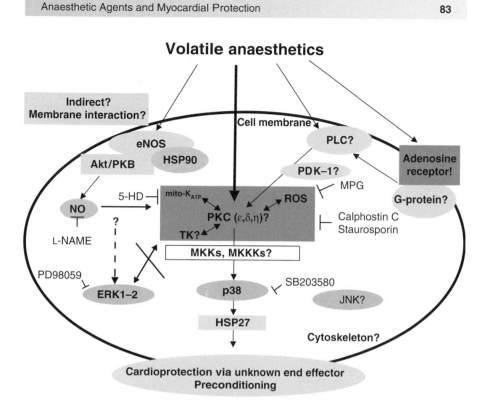

Figure 4.4 The mechanisms of anaesthetic preconditioning by the volatile agents are very complex and under constant investigation. The figure gives only a short overview. There are several different pathways involved in anaesthetic-induced preconditioning. Preconditioning by volatile anaesthetics involves the activation of PKC. The effect was shown by the use of specific PKC inhibitors: staurosporin and calphostin C. Also tyrosine kinases (TK) are discussed as mediators of cardioprotection by volatile anaesthetics, but their relationship to PKC is yet not defined. In addition, the family of MAP kinases (MAPK: p38, JNK and ERK) seems to be involved since the blockade by the specific inhibitors PD98059 (ERK1–2) and SB203580 (p38 MAPK) completely abolished the cardioprotection elicited by volatile anaesthetics. Whether the upstream kinases of MAPK, the MKKs and MKKKs are involved is poorly investigated and remains to be determined. Downstream of p38 MAPK, the phosphorylation of a member of the HSP family, HSP27, is upregulated resulting in cytoskeleton changes of the myocytes. The upstream signalling of PKC is yet not clearly defined. If the activation occurs via the PLC/3-PDK-1 pathway involving activation of G-protein-linked receptors or via opening of mito-K_{ATP} channels and release of ROS, or in parallel, has to be determined in detail. The role of mito-K_{ATP} has been extensively studied by the use of 5-HD, a specific blocker of the mito-K_{ATP} channels. Alternatively, it is suggested that the activation of eNOS, AKT (protein kinase B), HSP90 complex may lead to NO release and that this in turn activates K_{ATP} channels. A role for both NO and ROS in anaesthetic-induced preconditioning has been shown by the use of L-NAME, a specific NOS blocker, and MPG, a free-radical scavenger. The final steps to the still unknown end-effector mediating the protection by ischaemic and anaesthetic-induced preconditioning are still under investigation.

AKT (PKB): protein kinase B; eNOS: endothelial nitric oxide synthase; ERK1–2: extracellular signalling regulated kinases 1 and 2; 5-HD: 5-hydroxydecanoate, a blocker of mitochondrial K_{ATP}; mito-K_{ATP}: mitochondrial K_{ATP}; HSP: heat-shock protein; JNK: c-jun NH_2 terminal kinase; MKKs: MAPK kinases; MKKKs: MAPK kinase kinases; NO: nitric oxide; PDK: phosphatidylinositol trisphosphate-dependent kinase; PKC: protein kinase C; PLC: phospholipase C; ROS: reactive oxygen species, which are free oxygen radicals; TK: tyrosine kinase; Calphostin C and Staurosporin: blockers of PKC; L-NAME: NG-nitro-L-arginine methyl ester, a blocker of NO synthesis; MPG: N-(2-mercaptopropionyl)glycine, an intracellular oxygen radical scavenger; PD98059: blocker of ERK1–2.

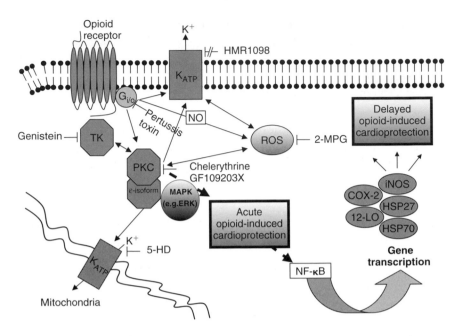

Figure 4.5 Schematic diagram of some of the major pathways which are thought to be involved in acute and delayed opioid-induced cardioprotection.

Acute opioid-induced cardioprotection: There are several different pathways involved in the acute phase of opioid-induced cardioprotection. After activation of the opioid receptor, there are at least two different pathways activated via $G_{i/o}$ proteins. (1) A micro-burst of reactive oxygen species (ROS), generated from intracellular nitric oxide (NO), leads to opening of sarcolemmal K_{ATP} (sarc-K_{ATP}). K_{ATP} opening generates additional ROS. (2) Protein kinase C (PKC) is activated, mainly the isoform ε is phosphorylated and translocated to the mitochondria. At the mitochondrial membrane, PKC-ε phosphorylates mitochondrial K_{ATP} (mito-K_{ATP}). Blocking mito-K_{ATP} with the specific antagonist 5-hydroxydecanoate (5-HD) abolishes acute opioid-induced cardioprotection, while blocking sarc-K_{ATP} with HMR1098 does not. Blocking tyrosine kinases (TK) with the unspecific blocking agent genistein abolishes the cardioprotective effect and prevents the activation of extracellular regulated kinases 1 and 2 (ERK1–2). Whether TK is downstream or parallel of PKC is currently not clear. If ROS are blocked via *N*-(2-mercaptopropionyl)glycine (MPG), cardioprotection is also abolished, demonstrating the central importance of ROS in acute opioid-induced cardioprotection.

Delayed opioid-induced cardioprotection: If PKC is activated via the above-described mechanism, MEK1 is activated and phosphorylates itself the 44 Da ERK (p44-ERK). Activation of the nuclear transcription factor κB (NF-κB) is thought to mediate the *de novo* synthesis of at least three mediators of delayed opioid-induced cardioprotection: the inducible isoform of NO synthase (iNOS), cyclo-oxygenase-2 (COX-2) and 12-lipo-oxygenase (12-LO). How these mediators promote cardioprotection remains unclear. Different from acute cardioprotection by opioids is the involvement of K_{ATP} channels. While the sarc-K_{ATP} is necessary during the trigger phase of delayed protection, the mito-K_{ATP} is important during the mediator phase.

provides an overview of a possible concept of the intracellular signal transduction of anaesthetic preconditioning.

Opioids can also stimulate preconditioning *in vitro* and *in vivo*. For opioid-induced preconditioning, an acute protective effect lasting for a few hours ('EPC') and delayed cardioprotection which reappears after 12–24 h and may last for a few days ('LPC') have been shown. Figure 4.5 provides an overview of our current understanding of intracellular signalling of opioid-induced cardioprotection. Unfortunately, opioid-induced preconditioning depends on activation of the δ_1-receptor, which is not activated by most of the clinically used opioids (except for morphine!). As species differences in signal transduction pathways may exist, it is reassuring that some of the key mechanisms of anaesthetic preconditioning (i.e. ATP-sensitive potassium (K_{ATP}) channel opening, adenosine receptor involvement, free radicals and mitogen-activated protein (MAP) kinases) have been confirmed in isolated human trabecula or myocardial cells.[26]

Potential Harmful Mechanisms: Blockade of Cardioprotection by Anaesthetics and Oral Hypoglycaemic Agents

Opening of the mitochondrial K_{ATP} channel is a central mechanism in the signal transduction of preconditioning (Fig. 4.3). Barbiturates and ketamine can block K_{ATP} channels in isolated cells. While thiopental appears to be safe and does not block experimental preconditioning at clinical doses,[27] several studies have found that ketamine completely blocks the cardioprotection of ischaemic preconditioning both *in vitro* and *in vivo*[28]; the effect is stereospecific for the $R(-)$-isomer. In experimental models, the substances propofol, etomidate, midazolam, dexmedetomidine and mivazerol had no effects on K_{ATP} channel activity.[29] While the clinical importance of these findings is still unknown, it is probably safer to avoid racemic ketamine in circumstances where ischaemia–reperfusion is likely to occur. Sulphonylurea oral hypoglycaemic drugs, such as glibenclamide, can block the K_{ATP} channel and prevent cardioprotection by preconditioning. Recent evidence suggests that a patient with Type II diabetes and coronary artery disease may benefit from changing the treatment to insulin (by having less ischaemia-induced myocardial dysfunction)[30].

Is anaesthetic-induced cardioprotection clinically relevant?

Several studies have shown a preconditioning effect for isoflurane,[31–33] enflurane[34] and sevoflurane.[35] However, all of the studies have examined relatively small groups ranging from 20 to 72 patients and, consequently, have had to use surrogate outcome markers such as post-ischaemic dysfunction and release of markers of cellular damage, for example troponins. Most studies have found better myocardial function (or less dysfunction)[34–36] and/or a decrease in myocardial injury markers.[31,33] Two of these studies also demonstrated an increase in biochemical markers indicating crucial signal transduction steps of preconditioning in biopsies of human myocardium[33,35]. With respect to protection against reperfusion injury, better post-bypass ventricular function and a decrease in troponin C release[15] were observed after short-term isoflurane treatment starting with the release of the aortic cross-clamp.

A more 'clinical' approach that probably combines the different protective mechanisms was used by De Hert and co-workers: they gave the volatile anaesthetic sevoflurane throughout the procedure (coronary artery bypass surgery) and compared patients anaesthetized using sevoflurane with patients anaesthetized with a total intravenous technique using propofol.[37] Although only 20 patients with good preoperative left ventricular function were enrolled in the study, they showed a marked difference in outcome: an improved ventricular function after termination of cardiopulmonary bypass in the sevoflurane group and less myocardial damage demonstrated by a markedly reduced troponin release in the following 26 h. These findings were confirmed in elderly patients with poor ventricular function[38] and the interim results from a multi-centre study by the same authors have also confirmed less troponin release with sevoflurane and desflurane anaesthesia compared with propofol or midazolam.[39]

Summary

In conclusion, there are strong cardioprotective mechanisms that can be influenced by anaesthetic agents. Anaesthetics may induce myocardial protection like the volatile anaesthetics (by preconditioning and by an action against reperfusion injury) or they may block protection mechanisms (like the blockade of preconditioning by racemic ketamine). From recent studies comes increasing evidence that cardioprotection by anaesthetic agents can be elicited in the clinical setting and may add to other organ protection strategies. Thus, it is conceivable that the choice of the anaesthetic drug may have an impact on patient outcome in ischaemia– reperfusion situations. However, this still has to be confirmed by large studies looking for definite outcome variables.

References

1. Spieckermann PG, Bruckner JB, Kübler W, Lohr B, Bretschneider HJ. Preischemic stress and resuscitation time of the heart. Verh Dtsch Ges Kreislaufforsch 1969; 33: 358–364.
2. Davis RF, DeBoer LW, Rude RE, Lowenstein E, Maroko PR. The effect of halothane anesthesia on myocardial necrosis, hemodynamic performance, and regional myocardial blood flow in dogs following coronary artery occlusion. Anesthesiology 1983; 59: 402–411.

3. Buljubasic N, Stowe DF, Marijic J, Roerig DL, Kampine JP, Bosnjak ZJ. Halothane reduces release of adenosine, inosine, and lactate with ischemia and reperfusion in isolated hearts. Anesth Analg 1993; 76: 54–62.
4. Buljubasic N, Marijic J, Stowe DF, Kampine JP, Bosnjak ZJ. Halothane reduces dysrhythmias and improves contractile function after global hypoperfusion in isolated hearts. Anesth Analg 1992; 74: 384–394.
5. Tarnow J, Markschies HA, Schulte SU. Isoflurane improves the tolerance to pacing-induced myocardial ischemia. Anesthesiology 1986; 64: 147–156.
6. Takahata O, Ichihara K, Ogawa H. Effects of sevoflurane on ischaemic myocardium in dogs. Acta Anaesthesiol Scand 1995; 39: 449–456.
7. Oguchi T, Kashimoto S, Yamaguchi T, Nakamura T, Kumazawa T. Comparative effects of halothane, enflurane, isoflurane and sevoflurane on function and metabolism in the ischaemic rat heart. Br J Anaesth 1995; 74: 569–575.
8. Pagel PS, Hettrick DA, Lowe D, Tessmer JP, Warltier DC. Desflurane and isoflurane exert modest beneficial actions on left ventricular diastolic function during myocardial ischemia in dogs. Anesthesiology 1995; 83: 1021–1035.
9. Rosenkranz ER, Buckberg GD. Myocardial protection during surgical coronary reperfusion. J Am Coll Cardiol 1983; 1: 1235–1246.
10. Braunwald E, Kloner RA. The stunned myocardium: prolonged, postischemic ventricular dysfunction. Circulation 1982; 66: 1146–1149.
11. Preckel B, Schlack W. Effect of anesthetics on ischemia–reperfusion injury of the heart. In: Vincent JL (ed.) 2002 Yearbook of Intensive Care and Emergency Medicine. Berlin: Springer, 2002; 165–176.
12. Schlack W, Hollmann M, Stunneck J, Thämer V. Effect of halothane on myocardial reoxygenation injury in the isolated rat heart. Br J Anaesth 1996; 76: 860–867.
13. Siegmund B, Schlack W, Ladilov YV, Piper HM. Halothane protects cardiomyocytes against reoxygenation-induced hypercontracture. Circulation 1997; 96: 4372–4379.
14. Kowalski C, Zahler S, Becker BF, Flaucher A, Conzen PF, Gerlach E et al. Halothane, isoflurane, and sevoflurane reduce postischemic adhesion of neutrophils in the coronary system. Anesthesiology 1997; 86: 188–195.
15. Buhre W. Cardioprotective and anti-inflammatory action of isoflurane during coronary artery bypass surgery. Habilitationsschrift RWTH Aachen 2001.
16. Ross S, Munoz H, Piriou V, Ryder WA, Foex P. A comparison of the effects of fentanyl and propofol on left ventricular contractility during myocardial stunning. Acta Anaesthesiol Scand 1998; 42: 23–31.
17. Ebel D, Schlack W, Comfère T, Preckel B, Thämer V. Effect of propofol on reperfusion injury after regional ischaemia in the isolated rat heart. Br J Anaesth 1999; 83: 903–908.
18. Murry CE, Jennings RB, Reimer KA. Preconditioning with ischemia: a delay of lethal cell injury in ischemic myocardium. Circulation 1986; 74: 1124–1136.
19. Qiu Y, Tang XL, Park SW, Sun JZ, Kalya A, Bolli R. The early and late phase of ischemic preconditioning. Circ Res 1997; 80: 730–742.
20. Yellon DM, Downey JM. Preconditioning the myocardium: from cellular physiology to clinical cardiology. Physiol Rev 2003; 83: 1113–1151.
21. Kloner RA, Shook T, Przyklenk K, Davis VG, Junio L, Matthews RV et al. Previous angina alters in-hospital outcome in TIMI 4. Circulation 1995; 91: 37–47.
22. Vaage J, Valen G. Preconditioning and cardiac surgery. Ann Thorac Surg 2003; 75: S709–S714.

23. Mullenheim J, Ebel D, Bauer M, Otto F, Heinen A, Frassdorf J *et al*. Sevoflurane confers additional cardioprotection after ischemic late preconditioning in rabbits. Anesthesiology 2003; 99: 624–631.

24. Toma O, Weber N, Obal D, Preckel B, Schlack W. Xenon induces myocardial protection by preconditioning. Involvement of protein kinase C (PKC). Anesthesiology 2003; 99: A1540.

25. Zaugg M, Lucchinetti E, Uecker M, Pasch T, Schaub MC. Anaesthetics and cardiac preconditioning. Part I. Signalling and cytoprotective mechanisms. Br J Anaesth 2003; 91: 551–565.

26. Tanaka K, Ludwig L, Kersten JR, Pagel PS, Warltier D. Mechanisms of cardioprotection by volatile anesthetics. Anesthesiology; in press.

27. Müllenheim J, Molojavyi A, Preckel B, Thämer V, Schlack W. Thiopentone does not block ischemic preconditioning in the isolated rat heart. Can J Anaesth 2001; 48: 784–789.

28. Müllenheim J, Fräßdorf J, Preckel B, Thämer V, Schlack W. Ketamine, but not S(+) blocks ischemia preconditioning in the rabbit heart in vivo. Anesthesiology 2001; 94: 630–636.

29. Zaugg M, Lucchinetti E, Garcia C, Pasch T, Spahn DR, Schaub MC. Anaesthetics and cardiac preconditioning. Part II. Clinical implications. Br J Anaesth 2003; 91: 566–576.

30. Scognamiglio R, Avogaro A, Vigili dK, Negut C, Palisi M, Bagolin E *et al*. Effects of treatment with sulfonylurea drugs or insulin on ischemia-induced myocardial dysfunction in type 2 diabetes. Diabetes 2002; 51: 808–812.

31. Tomai F, De Paulis R, Penta dP, Colagrande L, Caprara E, Polisca P *et al*. Beneficial impact of isoflurane during coronary bypass surgery on troponin I release. G Ital Cardiol 1999; 29: 1007–1014.

32. Haroun-Bizri S, Khoury SS, Chehab IR, Kassas CM, Baraka A. Does isoflurane optimize myocardial protection during cardiopulmonary bypass? J Cardiothorac Vasc Anesth 2001; 15: 418–421.

33. Belhomme D, Peynet J, Louzy M, Launay JM, Kitakaze M, Menasché P. Evidence for preconditioning by isoflurane in coronary artery bypass graft surgery. Circulation 1999; 100: 340–344.

34. Penta-de-Peppo A, Polisca P, Tomai F, De Paulis R, Turani F, Zupancich E *et al*. Recovery of LV contractility in man is enhanced by preischemic administration of enflurane. Ann Thorac surg 1999; 68: 112–118.

35. Julier K, da Silva R, Garcia C, Bestmann L, Frascarolo P, Zollinger A *et al*. Preconditioning by sevoflurane decreases biochemical markers for myocardial and renal dysfunction in coronary artery bypass graft surgery: a double-blinded, placebo-controlled, multicenter study. Anesthesiology 2003; 98: 1315–1327.

36. Haroun-Bizri S, Khoury SS, Chehab IR, Kassas CM, Baraka A. Does isoflurane optimize myocardial protection during cardiopulmonary bypass? J Cardiothorac Vasc Anesth 2001; 15: 418–421.

37. De Hert SG, ten Broecke PW, Mertens E, Van Sommeren EW, De Blier IG, Stockman BA *et al*. Sevoflurane but not propofol preserves myocardial function in coronary surgery patients. Anesthesiology 2002; 97: 42–49.

38. De Hert SG, Cromheecke S, ten Broecke PW, Mertens E, De Blier IG, Stockman BA *et al*. Effects of propofol, desflurane, and sevoflurane on recovery of myocardial function after coronary surgery in elderly high-risk patients. Anesthesiology 2003; 99: 314–323.

39. De Hert SG. Personal communication 2004.

R.S. Gardner   T.A. McDonagh

The treatment of heart failure due to left ventricular systolic dysfunction

This chapter aims to outline the management of both acute and chronic heart failure due to left ventricular systolic dysfunction. Before considering this in more detail, it is of paramount importance to realize that the best way to treat heart failure is to prevent it from happening in the first place. This should be by modifying known risk factors for ischaemic heart disease, and better treatment of myocardial infarction. An aetiology should always be sought for heart failure, as reversal of this may subsequently improve cardiac function. Once established heart failure has a poor prognosis, worse than many forms of cancer. The aims of treatment are, therefore, reduction in mortality and relief of symptoms. Indeed, recent advances in disease modifying therapy have markedly improved both morbidity and mortality.

Aetiology of Heart Failure

Causes of left ventricular systolic dysfunction include:

- Ischaemic heart disease.
- Valvular heart disease.
- Idiopathic (dilated cardiomyopathy).
- Hypertension.
- Alcohol excess.
- Viral (e.g. Coxsackie).
- Systemic disease (e.g. haemochromatosis, sarcoidosis, amyloidosis).

- Connective tissue disorders (e.g. systemic lupus erythematosus (systemic sclerosis).

- Neuromuscular disease (e.g. muscular dystrophy, Friedreich's ataxia).

- Glycogen storage disease (e.g. Pompe's disease).

- Cytotoxic drug therapy (e.g. doxorubicin, cyclophosphamide).

Epidemiology of Heart Failure

The incidence and prevalence of chronic heart failure increases with age and is greater in men than women. Approximately 3% of men and women aged 65–74 have chronic heart failure, rising to around 9% in the over 80s.[1] In a large epidemiological study in Glasgow, 2.9% of people aged 25–74 years had a significantly impaired left ventricular ejection fraction (≤30%), around half of whom were asymptomatic.[2] We may therefore have just discovered the tip of the iceberg in terms of the need for disease modifying therapy.

Pathophysiology of Heart Failure

The physiological definition of heart failure is not really of much use to the clinician ('an inability of the heart to provide sufficient oxygen to metabolizing tissues despite an adequate filling pressure'). In 1997, the European Society of Cardiology defined chronic heart failure as 'symptoms and signs of heart failure, and objective evidence of cardiac dysfunction, and where the diagnosis is in doubt, response to treatment directed towards heart failure'.[3]

Clinically, we know that heart failure is a syndrome, not a diagnosis; a syndrome comprising symptoms of breathlessness, fatigue and signs of fluid retention, and that heart failure develops secondary to chronic activation of the adrenergic and the renin–angiotensin–aldosterone systems, which leads to progressive cardiac dysfunction. Therefore, much of today's treatment for chronic heart failure is directed towards antagonism of these two systems.

Investigations

- Electrocardiogram (ECG) –abnormal in around 93% of cases. Common abnormalities include: evidence of previous myocardial infarction diffuse, non-specific ST segment and T wave changes, conduction abnormalities, sinus tachycardia and dysrhythmias (e.g. atrial fibrillation, ventricular ectopics, etc.).

- Chest X-ray – generalized cardiac enlargement. It may demonstrate pulmonary oedema.

- Echocardiogram – dilatation of the left ventricle and/or right ventricle with reduced systolic function – either global dysfunction (as in dilated cardiography) or a regional wall motion abnormality following myocardial infarction.

- Biochemistry and haematology.

- Coronary angiography to assess for potentially reversible causes of cardiac dysfunction.

- Nuclear imaging including radionuclide ventriculography.

- Progressive exercise test to quantify peak volume of oxygen consumption ($\dot{V}O_2$).

- Magnetic resonance imaging.

- Brain natriuretic peptide (BNP) – useful in both the diagnosis (strong negative predictive value) and assigning of prognosis in left ventricular systolic dysfunction.

Management of Chronic Heart Failure

Disease-modifying therapy

Angiotensin converting enzyme inhibitors
Angiotensin converting enzyme (ACE) inhibitors are first-line drugs which should be given to all patients with left ventricular systolic dysfunction, whether symptomatic[4,5] or not,[6] and should be combined with a diuretic if there is evidence of cardiac decompensation (e.g. peripheral or pulmonary oedema). The aggregate experience of a number of clinical trials involving more than 7000 patients has shown unequivocally that treatment with ACE inhibitors reduces both morbidity and mortality, with a 20–25% relative risk reduction on average. Unless there is a contraindication, such as significant renal disease, angioedema or an ACE inhibitor-induced cough, the use of ACE inhibitors in chronic heart failure should be considered mandatory.

β-blockers
Many studies have shown that β-blockers, including bisoprolol,[7] carvedilol[8–12] and metoprolol,[13] provide both a significant mortality reduction and long-term symptomatic benefit in patients with all grades of chronic heart failure, and in post-myocardial infarction left ventricular systolic dysfunction. It is imperative that β-blockers are started in patients who are free of cardiac decompensation and uptitrated slowly, 'start low, go slow'. Chronic obstructive airways disease without airways reversibility

and mild-to-moderate peripheral vascular disease should not be seen as contraindications to β-blocker therapy.

Aldosterone antagonists

Spironolactone has been shown to reduce mortality and morbidity in patients with moderate-to-severe chronic heart failure (New York Heart Association [NYHA] classes III and IV), when used in addition to standard therapy (ACE inhibitor and β-blocker).[14] More recently, eplerenone has been shown to have similar effects in post-myocardial infarction left ventricular systolic dysfunction.[15] However, caution should be exercised with these drugs as they can impair renal function and cause significant hyperkalaemia.

Angiotensin II receptor antagonists

Angiotensin II receptor antagonists have been shown to be an effective alternative in truly ACE intolerant individuals, although ACE inhibitors should be regarded as the first-line drugs of choice. In the recent Candesartan in Heart Failure-Assessment of Reduction in Mortality and Morbidity (CHARM) study, however, the addition of candesartan to existing triple therapy (ACE inhibitor [100%], β-blocker [55%] and spironolactone [17%]) reduced cardiovascular death and hospitalization for chronic heart failure by 15%.[16] This trial suggested that patients remaining symptomatic despite ACE inhibitor and β-blocker, may now have another therapeutic option.

Hydralazine and nitrates

Hydralazine and nitrates can also be considered in patients intolerant to both ACE inhibitors and Angiotensin receptor antagonists.[17,18]

Symptomatic therapy

Diuretics

Diuretics still have an important place in the management of both the symptoms and signs of fluid retention in chronic heart failure. It should be remembered that diuretics have not been shown to confer a mortality benefit and indeed higher doses are associated with a worse outcome.[19,20] Therefore, as low a diuretic dose as possible should be used along with a fluid restriction if necessary. Usually a loop diuretic, such as frusemide or bumetamide is necessary. Once doses of frusemide of 160 mg/day are reached, sequential nephron blockade with a thiazide diuretic (e.g. bendrofluazide or metolazone) may relieve signs of fluid retention with more efficacy than further increases in the loop diuretic dose. Renal function should be monitored closely and hypokalaemia corrected.

Digoxin

The role of digoxin appears less clear. The current recommendations are for this drug to be introduced in patients who remain symptomatic despite maximal medical therapy, or to provide rate control to patients with atrial fibrillation. In two large studies with digoxin,[21,22] however, patients with atrial fibrillation were excluded, and no mortality benefit was demonstrated. Indeed, post-hoc analyses of the Digitalis Investigation Group (DIG) trial has shown that female subjects on digoxin had a higher mortality than those not on digoxin,[23] and in another study male subjects with higher serum digoxin concentrations (>1.2 ng/ml) had a higher mortality than patients receiving placebo.[24] Digoxin is best reserved for patients who remain very symptomatic, with large hearts and frequent hospitalizations. Digoxin therapy should be avoided in those with ventricular dysrhythmias.

Other pharmacological therapy

Patients with ischaemic heart disease should be prescribed aspirin unless there is a specific contraindication. The benefits of warfarin therapy in chronic heart failure are currently uncertain, except in patients with atrial fibrillation or known left ventricular thrombus, and this was the subject of two large clinical trials in chronic heart failure (WATCH and WASH). Statin therapy has been shown to be of benefit in both primary and secondary prevention in ischaemic heart disease, but there has been recent debate as to the safety of statins in chronic heart failure. A recent report however suggests that statin therapy may reduce mortality significantly in non-ischaemic NYHA classes III/IV chronic heart failure.[25] It has also been suggested that long-term use of high-dose allopurinol could be associated with a reduced mortality, possibly by negating the adverse effect of an elevated urate concentration.[26] Clinical trials to address this question are now ongoing.

Anaemia is common in chronic heart failure and has been shown to be an independent predictor of mortality.[27] Initial reports have demonstrated a reduction in hospital admissions and improvement in cardiac function in patients with moderate-to-severe chronic heart failure treated with erythropoietin and intravenous iron,[28] and larger studies are currently under way. Furthermore it is important to avoid, if possible, drugs that may exacerbate chronic heart failure (e.g. non-steroidal anti-inflammatory drugs (NSAIDs), rate-limiting calcium antagonists (diltiazem and verapamil), class I anti-arrhythmic drugs, steroids and tricyclic anti-depressants).

Non-pharmacological intervention and lifestyle modification

Lifestyle modifications should be encouraged, for example cessation of smoking and alcohol (especially if this is thought to be the aetiology),[29] weight loss (where appropriate) and engagement in aerobic exercise, if possible.[30] Annual immunization for influenza and pneumococcus is recommended.[31] Fluid restriction of between 1l and 2 l/day should be employed and the patient counselled in the importance of monitoring their fluid balance, by for example daily weighing. Salt rich foods should also be avoided.

Device therapy

Automatic implantable cardioverter defibrillators (AICDs)

Following the publication of the Multicenter Automatic Defibrillator Implantation Trial (MADIT) II study,[32] it is clear that patients with left ventricular systolic dysfunction secondary to ischaemic heart disease with a left ventricular ejection fraction <35%, benefit in terms of mortality reduction from automatic implantable cardioverter defibrillator (AICD) implantation. Implementation of this has significant cost implications. Currently AICDs are implanted into patients with ischaemic heart disease and left ventricular systolic dysfunction with ventricular dysrhythmias.

Cardiac resynchronization therapy (CRT)

Cardiac resynchronization therapy (CRT) is the subject of much research in chronic heart failure. In combination with stable, optimal medical therapy, CRT may improve the well-being of the patient by correcting ventricular dysynchrony. This is achieved by the insertion of pacing leads into the right atrium and right ventricle as with a standard dual chamber (DDD) pacemaker, but also by pacing the left ventricle via a lead placed in the coronary sinus. This is known to improve symptoms, reduce hospitalizations, increase effort capacity and improve haemodynamics in patients in NYHA classes III/IV with wide QRS complexes. Its effects on mortality are unknown and currently being studied in the CARE-heart failure trial.[33] Combined CRT/AICD implantation does reduce mortality in chronic heart failure Comparison of Medical Therapy, Pacing, and Defibrillation in Heart Failure Trial (COMPANION trial).[34,35] The place of CRT alone in chronic heart failure remains to be determined.

Left ventricular assist devices

Left ventricular assist devices (LVADs) are blood pumps that take over part of the heart's pumping function when implanted alongside or within the heart. They are now emerging as treatment options in advanced heart failure either as a bridge to transplantation, a bridge to recovery or as destination therapy (for patients with end-stage heart failure who require permanent mechanical heart support and are not suitable for cardiac transplantation).[36]

Surgical options

In patients who fail to respond to medical or device therapy, surgical options include revascularization for hibernating myocardium, ventricular remodelling (less commonly performed now), and cardiac transplantation.

Cardiac transplantation

Although donor organ availability restricts its use, cardiac transplantation remains an option for those patients with advanced heart failure who fail to respond to medical therapy. It carries a significant 1-year mortality of around 19% and an average life expectancy of 10 years.[37] Although patients are required to have severe left ventricular systolic dysfunction to warrant this procedure, due to the impact of major surgery and the significant side effects of the immunosuppressive regimen, they must otherwise be well.

Management of Acute Heart Failure

Much less is known about the management of acute heart failure than chronic. Part of the problem is the heterogeneous nature of acute heart failure, which masquerades under numerous titles including 'acute heart failure', 'exacerbation of heart failure' and 'decompensated heart failure.' By acute heart failure we normally mean a sudden onset of symptoms or signs of heart failure in a patient with no history of heart failure and previously normal cardiac function. This usually occurs secondary to either acute myocardial infarction, with or without its mechanical sequelae, or fulminant myocarditis. The treatment has to be aimed at the underlying condition as well as the heart failure. This condition has a highly variable prognosis and represents only a small minority of hospitalized heart failure patients. In contrast decompensated heart failure and exacerbation of heart failure occur in patients with an established diagnosis of heart failure where they experience increasing symptoms or signs of heart failure after a period of stability. This constitutes the majority of hospitalizations for heart failure, and is particularly relevant to the anaesthetist when considering fluid balance pre-, peri- and postoperatively.

The management of acute heart failure has essentially remained unchanged for decades and is only now becoming widely investigated. Treatment largely consists of intravenous loop diuretics and opiates for the relief of the symptoms and signs of acute pulmonary oedema, principally by vasodilatation and reduction in preload. In addition intravenous nitrates have proven efficacy.[38] However, intravenous use of the latter agents is often hampered by tolerance to them after the first 24 h and may also lead to significant arterial hypotension which results in reduced renal perfusion and a poor diuretic response. If this occurs it is then often necessary to employ intravenous inotropes to augment the blood pressure.

In acute heart failure where there are already high circulating concentrations of endogenous catecholamines, dobutamine may also be used. There are no randomized controlled trials comparing dobutamine with placebo and many clinicians contend that dobutamine is potentially harmful and associated with an adverse mortality. Alternatives to dobutamine include the phosphodiesterase inhibitors milrinone and enoximone which work via an action on non-cyclic AMP-mediated pathways. Milrinone was associated with a trend to an increase in adverse events in the Outcomes of a Prospective Trial of Intravenous Milrinone for Exacerbations of chronic heart failure (OPTIME-CHF) trial; the largest acute heart failure trial which involved 949 patients.[39] There have been no studies of the use of enoximone in acute heart failure. Although dopamine has in the past been used to improve renal perfusion in oliguric patients with acute heart failure, it has never been subject to a randomized control trial in this patient population. Its use is, at best, highly contentious.

Recent advances in the therapy of acute heart failure

Nesiritide (human recombinant B-type natriuretic peptide; BNP) principally causes vasodilatation by increasing cGMP, thus lowering left ventricular filling pressures. Investigators in the Vasodilatation in the Management of ACute heart failure (VMAC) study compared the use of intravenous nesiritide with intravenous glyceryl trinitrate (GTN) and found that BNP reduced pulmonary capillary wedge pressure more effectively than GTN, and was associated with an earlier improvement in symptoms of breathlessness.[40,41] However, the 30-day rehospitalization rates were similar between the two groups and there was no significant difference in 6-month mortality rates in patients receiving nesiritide compared with GTN (25.1% and 20.8%, respectively). Nesiritide has also been compared with dobutamine in patients with acute decompensated heart failure. Patients treated with nesiritide were found to have a reduced mortality when compared to patients treated with dobutamine.[42] In addition, nesiritide caused fewer dysrhythmias.[43]

Levosimendan is an inodilator, which acts by increasing the sensitivity of troponin-C to intracellular calcium, as well vasodilatation through vascular

K-ATPase channels. The recent Levosimendan infusion versus Dobutamine in Severe Low Output Heart Failure (LIDO) study reported a beneficial effect of levosimendan on haemodynamic performance and a lower mortality rate than with dobutamine in low-output heart failure.[44] The findings of the LIDO study were reinforced by similar findings in post cardiogenic shock patients in the Randomized Study on Safety and Effectiveness of Levosimendan in Patients with Left Ventricular Failure After an Acute Myocardial Infarct (RUSSLAN) trial, where levosimendan was compared with placebo.[45]

Non-invasive ventilation

Non-invasive ventilation has recently been shown to improve symptoms in acute heart failure.[46] In acute pulmonary oedema, continuous positive airway pressure (CPAP) theoretically limits the decrease in functional residual capacity, improves respiratory haemodynamics and oxygenation, and decreases left ventricular afterload, thus leading to a more rapid clinical recovery. However, the widespread use of this ventilatory technique is not currently recommended by major clinical guidelines.[3,47] In a multicentre study, patients with cardiogenic pulmonary oedema were randomized to receive either medical therapy plus oxygen, or non-invasive pressure support ventilation.[48] The latter group had a significantly faster improvement in partial pressure of oxygen/fraction of inspired oxygen (P_aO_2/F_iO_2), respiratory rate and dyspnoea, although the intubation rate, hospital mortality and length of hospital stay were similar in the two groups. However, in the subgroup of patients with hypercapnia (partial pressure of carbon dioxide, $P_aCO_2 > 6\,kPa$ [45 mmHg]) non-invasive pressure support ventilation improved P_aCO_2 significantly faster and reduced the intubation rate more when compared with medical therapy. Invasive ventilation using intermittent positive pressure ventilation can also be helpful in extreme cases where the patient is incapable of maintaining adequate oxygen saturation while self-ventilating.

Summary

Until recently, the goal for the treatment of heart failure was to relieve symptoms and enhance functional capacity. However, studies have now shown that treatment with ACE inhibitors and β adrenergic receptor blockade can reduce both the morbidity and the mortality of chronic heart failure. In addition cardiac resynchronization therapy when combined with AICD implantation also reduces mortality in chronic heart failure. In acute heart failure there is increasing evidence that treatment with human recombinant B-type natriuretic peptide (nesiritide) and levosimendan is associated with reduced mortality when compared with conventional treatment with dobutamine.

The findings of the Calcium Sensitizer or Inotrope or None in Low Output Heart Failure study (CASINO) study have revealed a clear advantage for levosimendan over conventional treatment for acute heart failure. The study, which was designed to evaluate the efficacy of levosimendan therapy in patients with decompensated heart failure (but unlike previous studies included a placebo group), was halted prematurely because the 6-month mortality in dobutamine-treated patients was significantly higher than the 6-month mortality in levosimendan and placebo-treated patients (39.6% versus 15.3% versus 24.7%; American College of Cardiology 53rd Annual Scientific Session 2004; Abstract 835–836).

The results of the CASINO study and other recent clinical trials are outlined in Cleland JG, Ghosh J, Freemantle N *et al*. Clinical trials update and cumulative meta-analyses from the American College of Cardiology: WATCH, SCD-HeFT, DINAMIT, CASINO, INSPIRE, STRATUS-US, RIO-Lipids and cardiac resynchronization therapy in heart failure. Eur J Heart Fail 2004; 6: 501–508.

References

1. McKee PA, Castelli WP, McNamara PM, Kannel WB. The natural history of congestive heart failure: the Framingham Study. New Engl J Med 1971; 285: 1441–1446.
2. McDonagh TA, Morrison CE, Lawrence A *et al*. Symptomatic and asymptomatic left-ventricular systolic dysfunction in an urban population. Lancet 1997; 350: 829–833.
3. The treatment of heart failure. Task Force of the Working Group on Heart Failure of the European Society of Cardiology. Eur Heart J 1997; 18: 736–753.
4. The SOLVD Investigators. Effect of enalapril on survival in patients with reduced left ventricular ejection fractions and congestive heart failure. New Engl J Med 1991; 325: 293–302.
5. Swedberg K, IdanpaanHeikkila U, Remes J *et al*. Effects of enalapril on mortality in severe congestive heart failure. Results of the COoperative North Scandinavian ENalapril SUrvival Study (CONSENSUS). New Engl J Med 1987; 316: 1429–1435.
6. The SOLVD Investigators. Effect of enalapril on mortality and the development of heart failure in asymptomatic patients with reduced left ventricular ejection fractions. [published erratum appears in New Engl J Med 1992; 10; 327: 1768] New Engl J Med 1992; 327: 685–691.
7. Anonymous. The Cardiac Insufficiency BIsoprolol Study II (CIBIS-II): a randomised trial. Lancet 1999; 353: 9–13.
8. Packer M, Coats AJ, Fowler MB *et al*. Effect of carvedilol on survival in severe chronic heart failure. New Engl J Med 2001; 344: 1651–1658.

9. Packer M, Bristow MR, Cohn JN et al. The effect of carvedilol on morbidity and mortality in patients with chronic heart failure. U.S. Carvedilol Heart failure Study Group. New Engl J Med 1996; 334: 1349–1355.

10. Olsen SL, Gilbert EM, Renlund DG, Taylor DO, Yanowitz FD, Bristow MR. Carvedilol improves left ventricular function and symptoms in chronic heart failure: a double-blind randomized study. J Am Coll Cardiol 1995; 25: 1225–1231.

11. Anonymous. Effects of carvedilol, a vasodilator-beta-blocker, in patients with congestive heart failure due to ischemic heart disease. Australia–New Zealand Heart failure Research Collaborative Group. Circulation 1995; 92: 212–218.

12. Bristow MR, Gilbert EM, Abraham WT et al. Carvedilol produces dose-related improvements in left ventricular function and survival in subjects with chronic heart failure. Circulation 1996; 94: 2807–2816.

13. Anonymous. Effect of metoprolol CR/XL in chronic heart failure: MEtoprolol CR/XL Randomised Intervention Trial in congestive Heart Failure (MERIT-HF). Lancet 1999; 353: 2001–2007.

14. Pitt B, Zannad F, Remme WJ, Cody R, Castaigne A, Perez A et al. The effect of spironolactone on morbidity and mortality in patients with severe heart failure. Randomized Aldactone Evaluation Study Investigators. New Engl J Med 1999; 341: 709–717.

15. Pitt B, Remme W, Zannad F, Neaton J, Martinez F, Roniker B, Bittman R, Hurley S, Kleiman J, Gatlin M, and the Eplerenone Post-Acute Myocardial Infarction Heart Failure Efficacy and Survival Study Investigators. Eplerenone, a selective aldosterone blocker, in patients with left ventricular dysfunction after myocardial infarction. New Eng J Med 2003; 348: 1309–1321.

16. McMurray JJV, Ostergren J, Swedberg K, Granger CB, Held P, Michelson EL, Olofsson B, Yusuf S, Pfeffer MA. Effects of candesartan in patients with chronic heart failure and reduced left-ventricular systolic function taking angiotensin-converting-enzyme inhibitors: the CHARM-added trial. Lancet 2003; 362: 767–771.

17. Cohn JN, Johnson G, Ziesche S et al. A comparison of enalapril with hydralazine-isosorbide dinitrate in the treatment of patients with chronic congestive heart failure. New Engl J Med 1991; 325: 303–310.

18. Cohn JN, Archibald DG, Ziesche S et al. Effect of vasodilator therapy on mortality in chronic congestive heart failure: results of a veterans administration cooperative study. New Engl J Med 1986; 314: 1547–1552.

19. Neuberg GW, Miller AB, O'Connor CM et al. Diuretic resistance predicts mortality in patients with advanced heart failure. Am Heart J 2002; 144: 31–38.

20. Batin P, Wickens M, McEntegart D, Fullwood L, Cowley AJ. The importance of abnormalities of liver function tests in predicting mortality in chronic heart failure. Eur Heart J 1995; 16: 1613–1618.

21. Anonymous. The effect of digoxin on mortality and morbidity in patients with heart failure. The Digitalis Investigation Group. New Engl J Med 1997; 336: 525–533.

22. Packer M, Gheorghiade M, Young JB, Costantini PJ, Adams KF, Cody RJ et al. Withdrawal of digoxin from patients with chronic heart failure treated with angiotensin-converting-enzyme inhibitors. RADIANCE Study. New Engl J Med 1993; 329: 1–7.

23. Rathore SS, Wang Y, Krumholz HM. Sex-based differences in the effect of digoxin for the treatment of heart failure. New Engl J Med 2002; 347: 1403–1411.

24. Rathore SS, Curtis JP, Wang Y, Bristow MR, Krumholz HM. Association of serum digoxin concentration and outcomes in patients with heart failure. J Am Med Assoc 2003; 289: 871–878.
25. Anker SD, Clark AL, Kilowski C et al. Statins and survival in 2068 HF patients with ischemic and non-ischemic etiology. Circulation 2002; 106: 2535A.
26. Struthers AD, Donnan PT, Lindsay P et al. Effect of allopurinol on mortality and hospitalisations in chronic heart failure: a retrospective cohort study. Heart 2002; 87: 229–234.
27. Ezekowitz JA, McAlister FA, Armstrong PW. Anemia is common in heart failure and is associated with poor outcomes: insights from a cohort of 12065 patients with new-onset heart failure. Circulation 2003; 107: 223–225.
28. Silverberg DS, Wexler D, Sheps D et al. The effect of correction of mild anemia in severe, resistant congestive heart failure using subcutaneous erythropoietin and intravenous iron: a randomized controlled study. J Am Coll Cardiol 2001; 37: 1775–1780.
29. Guillo P, Mansourati J, Maheu B et al. Long-term prognosis in patients with alcoholic cardiomyopathy and severe heart failure after total abstinence. Am J Cardiol 1997; 79: 1276–1278.
30. Belardinelli R, Georgiou D, Cianci G, Purcaro A. Randomized, controlled trial of long-term moderate exercise training in chronic heart failure: effects on functional capacity, quality of life, and clinical outcome [see comments]. Circulation 1999; 99: 1173–1182.
31. Opasich C, Febo O, Riccardi PG et al. Concomitant factors of decompensation in chronic heart failure. Am J Cardiol 1996; 78: 354–357.
32. Moss AJ, Hall WJ, Cannom DS et al. Improved survival with an implanted defibrillator in patients with coronary disease at high risk for ventricular arrhythmia. New Engl J Med 1996; 335: 1933–1940.
33. Cleland JG, Daubert JC, Erdmann E et al. The CARE-Heart Failure Study (CArdiac REsynchronisation in Heart Failure Study): rationale, design and endpoints. Eur J Heart Fail 2001; 3: 481–489.
34. Bristow MR, Feldman AM, Saxon LA. Heart failure management using implantable devices for ventricular resynchronization: comparison of medical therapy, pacing, and defibrillation in chronic heart failure (COMPANION) trial. COMPANION Steering Committee and COMPANION Clinical Investigators. J Cardiac Fail 2000; 6: 276–285.
35. Feldman AM, Bristow MR. The comparison of medical therapy, pacing and defibrillation in heart failure (COMPANION) trial. American College of Cardiology Scientific Sessions 2003.
36. Aaronson KD, Patel H, Pagani FD. Patient selection for left ventricular assist device therapy. Ann Thorac Surg 2003; 75(Suppl 6): S29–S35.
37. Hosenpud JD, Bennet LE, Keck BM, Boucek MM, Novick RJ. ISHLT Registry Report: the registry of the international society for heart and lung transplantation: Seventeenth Official Report-2000. J Heart Lung Transplant 2000; 19: 909–931.
38. Northridge D. Frusemide or nitrates for acute heart failure? Lancet 1996; 347: 667–668.
39. Cuffe MS, Califf RM, Adams Jr KF et al. Outcomes of a Prospective Trial of Intravenous Milrinone for Exacerbations of Chronic Heart Failure (OPTIME-CHF) investigators. Short term intravenous milrinone for acute exacerbation of chronic heart failure: a randomized control trial. J Am Med Assoc 2002; 287: 1541–1547.

40. Publication Committee for the VMAC Investigators (Vasodilatation in the Management of ACute heart failure). Intravenous nesiritide vs nitroglycerin for the treatment of decompensated congestive heart failure: a randomised control trial. J Am Med Assoc 2002; 39: 1531–1540.

41. Colucci WS, Elkayam U, Horton DP, Abraham WT, Bourge RC, Johnson AD *et al.* Intravenous nesiritide, a natriuretic peptide, in the treatment of decompensated congestive heart failure. Nesiritide Study Group. New Engl J Med 2000; 343: 246–253.

42. Silver MA, Horton DP, Ghali JK, Elkayam U. Effect of nesiritide versus dobutamine on short-term outcomes in the treatment of patients with acutely decompensated heart failure. J Am Coll Cardiol 2002; 39: 798–803.

43. Burger AJ, Elkayam U, Neibaur MT *et al.* Comparison of the occurrence of ventricular arrhythmias in patients with acutely decompensated congestive heart failure receiving dobutamine versus nesiritide therapy. Am J Cardiol 2001; 88: 35–39.

44. Follath F, Cleland JG, Just H *et al.* Efficacy and safety of intravenous levosimendan compared with dobutamine in severe low-output heart failure (the LIDO Study): a randomised double-blind trial. Lancet 2002; 360: 196–202.

45. Moiseyev VS, Poder P, Andrejevs N *et al.* Safety and efficacy of a novel calcium sensitizer, levosimendan, in patients with left ventricular failure due to an acute myocardial infarction. A randomized, placebo-controlled, double-blind study (RUSSLAN). Eur Heart J 2002; 23: 1422–1432.

46. Panacek EA, Kirk JD. Role of noninvasive ventilation in the management of acutely decompensated heart failure. Rev Cardiovasc Med 2002; 3(Suppl): S35–S40.

47. Guidelines for the evaluation and management of heart failure. Report of the American College of Cardiology/American Heart Association Task Force on Practice Guidelines (Committee on Evaluation and Management of Heart failure). J Am Coll Cardiol 1995; 26: 1376–1398.

48. Nava S, Carbone G, DiBattista N *et al.* Noninvasive ventilation in cardiogenic pulmonary oedema: a multicenter randomized trial. Am J Resp Crit Care Med 2003; 168: 1432–1437.

A.R. Edouard   V. Minville   L. Martin

Blunt chest trauma

Chest trauma accounts for approximately 20–25% of traumatic deaths.[1] The majority of thoracic injuries occur as a result of blunt trauma. Life-threatening situations may result from apparently minor trauma mainly due to the presence of major organs in the thorax, and of the large body surface involved in the injury. Cardiorespiratory failure is usually related to missed chest injuries and delayed treatment.[2]

The classification of thoracic injuries is presented here according to the 'Organ Injury Scale', focusing mainly on the functional consequences of chest wall, pulmonary, and cardiovascular injuries. Since a rapid identification of cardiorespiratory failure and a prompt diagnosis of chest injuries are needed, some clinical management guidelines are proposed, taking into account the newer imaging technology, especially bedside ultrasonography and multislice computerized tomography (CT), even though these practices are not always evidently based.[2] Finally, specific therapeutic propositions are considered for the management of patients with blunt chest trauma.

Chest Injuries and Functional Consequences

Chest injuries are often associated with head and abdominal injuries. Major thoracic injuries can occur without clear external damage, and obvious extrathoracic injuries can delay the diagnosis of chest trauma. Thoracic injuries may result from either direct trauma (blunt or crush) or indirect trauma (deceleration or blast).

Cardiorespiratory failure

Blunt chest trauma has a combined effect on respiratory and haemodynamic functions. The consequences of chest trauma are rapidly associated with the adverse effect of other injuries. Hypoxaemia may be related to hypovolaemia through the blood loss of a haemothorax, to ventilation–perfusion mismatch due to lung contusion or lung collapse, and to changes in intrathoracic pressure related to a tension pneumothorax. Acidosis can be of metabolic or respiratory origin. The former derives from tissue hypoperfusion and the latter is due to inadequate ventilation, which in this case is related to airway injury, altered level of consciousness and intrathoracic pressure changes. Circulatory failure is usually related to hypovolaemia, but may also be caused by a restriction of cardiac filling by pleural or pericardial effusion. Furthermore, ventricular dysrhythmias or myocardial dysfunction due to myocardial contusion may be the significant contributive factors.

Chest injuries

Organ Injury Scaling measures injury severity scores for individual organs to facilitate clinical research and provides an initial classification system. The grading scheme is fundamentally an anatomical description, ranging from 1 to 5, representing the least and the most severe injury, respectively. A level of ⩾3 corresponds to significant chest trauma. Chest wall, lung, heart, thoracic vessels, and diaphragm are taken into account in the Organ Injury Scale (Fig. 6.1).[3]

Chest wall injuries

Rib fractures occur in 50–70% of patients with blunt chest trauma. Flail chest is observed in 5–13% of the patients.[1] Flail chest is defined by the fracture of three or more adjacent ribs at two or more points, such that the involved segment can move independently and paradoxically from the remaining chest wall. The magnitude of this paradoxical movement of the chest wall contributes to the severity of respiratory failure. The main cause of hypoxaemia is the accompanying pulmonary contusion. Pain can be due to periostial lengthening, intercostal nerve stimulation, or pleural injury. Gastric distention and muscle spasm are direct consequences of pain. An increase in the work of breathing is usually observed between the second and the third post-traumatic day.

Sternal and scapular fractures.   These are direct evidence of a violent impact but do not have an intrinsic prognostic value as compared with the number of fractured ribs.[4–6] Conversely, injuries of the adjacent nervous and vascular structures are more frequent when the first or second ribs are

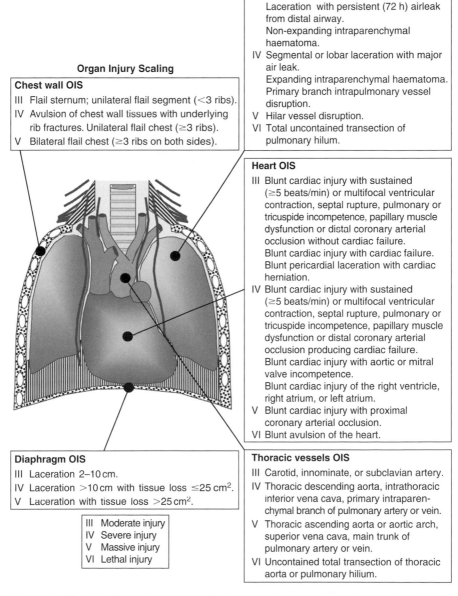

Organ Injury Scaling

Lung OIS

III Unilateral contusion (1 lobe)
Laceration with persistent (72 h) airleak from distal airway.
Non-expanding intraparenchymal haematoma.

IV Segmental or lobar laceration with major air leak.
Expanding intraparenchymal haematoma.
Primary branch intrapulmonary vessel disruption.

V Hilar vessel disruption.

VI Total uncontained transection of pulmonary hilum.

Chest wall OIS

III Flail sternum; unilateral flail segment (<3 ribs).

IV Avulsion of chest wall tissues with underlying rib fractures. Unilateral flail chest (≥3 ribs).

V Bilateral flail chest (≥3 ribs on both sides).

Heart OIS

III Blunt cardiac injury with sustained (≥5 beats/min) or multifocal ventricular contraction, septal rupture, pulmonary or tricuspide incompetence, papillary muscle dysfunction or distal coronary arterial occlusion without cardiac failure.
Blunt cardiac injury with cardiac failure.
Blunt pericardial laceration with cardiac herniation.

IV Blunt cardiac injury with sustained (≥5 beats/min) or multifocal ventricular contraction, septal rupture, pulmonary or tricuspide incompetence, papillary muscle dysfunction or distal coronary arterial occlusion producing cardiac failure.
Blunt cardiac injury with aortic or mitral valve incompetence.
Blunt cardiac injury of the right ventricle, right atrium, or left atrium.

V Blunt cardiac injury with proximal coronary arterial occlusion.

VI Blunt avulsion of the heart.

Diaphragm OIS

III Laceration 2–10 cm.

IV Laceration >10 cm with tissue loss ≤25 cm².

V Laceration with tissue loss >25 cm².

III	Moderate injury
IV	Severe injury
V	Massive injury
VI	Lethal injury

Thoracic vessels OIS

III Carotid, innominate, or subclavian artery.

IV Thoracic descending aorta, intrathoracic inferior vena cava, primary intraparen-chymal branch of pulmonary artery or vein.

V Thoracic ascending aorta or aortic arch, superior vena cava, main trunk of pulmonary artery or vein.

VI Uncontained total transection of thoracic aorta or pulmonary hilium.

Figure 6.1 Classification of the thoracic injuries according to the Organ Injury Scaling (OIS).

fractured because of the narrow thoracic inlet and the magnitude of the trauma necessarily involved.[4]

Diaphragmatic injury. Diaphragmatic injury is observed in 7% of patients with blunt chest trauma. Large radial tears of the diaphragm are more frequent on the left side,[7] and are commonly associated with intrathoracic and extrathoracic visceral injuries[1] with or without herniation of the abdominal viscera. Diaphragmatic dysfunction may occur in one-third of the patients with blunt chest trauma in the absence of anatomical injury and lasts several weeks.

Pulmonary injuries

Lung contusion.   Lung contusion is defined as a disruption of alveolar capillary integrity resulting in intra-alveolar haemorrhage and oedema, is observed in 17–26% of patients in the vicinity of costal, sternal, or vertebral fractures.[8] Contusion has to be differentiated from post-traumatic atelectasis related to mechanical ventilation, from inhalation of gastric content or blood, or from lung collapse due to compression by pneumothorax or haemothorax. Reduced surfactant production associated with lung contusion induces a decrease in parenchymal compliance, leading to ventilation–perfusion mismatch. Lung contusion is a source of circulating inflammatory mediators which cause a regional capillary leak, affecting non-traumatized areas of the lung.[9] Aggressive fluid resuscitation with crystalloids may predispose to acute lung injury and pulmonary infection.[10,11] Contusion is also complicated by acute lung injury in 30–80% of patients.[12,13] Lung contusion is therefore an evolving disease with a peak of deleterious consequences between the first and the second post-traumatic day.[12,14] The need for ventilatory support is related to the extent of the initial injury and the evolution of the lung damage.[8,12] Pulmonary contusion, rather than chest wall injury is the main cause of long-term respiratory dysfunction resulting in a decreased functional residual capacity.[15]

Pneumothorax.   Pneumothorax is observed in 20% of patients with blunt chest trauma.[1] It is usually related to a cortical tear or a very distal airway injury and is frequently limited to the anterior part of the pleural cavity. Bilateral pneumothoraces are only observed in 10% of patients.[16] The degree of associated lung contusion and pneumothorax depends on the severity of the lung injury: 14% for minor contusion rising to 63% for pulmonary lacerations.[8,12] Tension pneumothorax occurs in 10% of patients with pneumothorax. It may hinder ventilation on the contralateral side and reduces venous return to the heart.

Tracheal and bronchial wounds.   These are rare and only affect 0.3% of patients with blunt chest trauma.[17] Transection of the trachea or bronchi proximal to the pleural reflection cause extensive mediastinal, cervical, and subcutaneous emphysema. Injuries distal to the pleural reflection result in pneumothoraces. Haemoptysis, tension pneumothorax, and persisting air leak are signs of bronchial injury.

Haemothorax.   The source of pleural bleeding is usually the chest wall (rib fractures and intercostal vessels) or pulmonary surface. Massive haemothorax is defined by a blood loss of >1500 ml into the chest cavity. Such extensive bleeding suggests a direct damage to the hilar structures, the large vessels, or the heart.

Cardiovascular injuries

Myocardial contusion.   Myocardial contusion occurs in about 15% of patients with blunt chest trauma.[18] Myocardial contusion or blunt cardiac injury is characterized by haemorrhagic infiltrate, tissue oedema, and bands, usually observed in the anterior, apical, or basal part of the heart depending on the type of impact (direct thoracic impact, increase in abdominal pressure).[19] Myocardial injuries can be related to trauma impact and/or to a forced ventricular contraction,[20] thus explaining the abnormal movement of the wall and the release of necrosis markers. This may be observed with or without chest trauma[21] and electrocardiograph (ECG) abnormalities.[22]

Cardiovascular complications.   Cardiovascular complications of myocardial contusion are observed in up to 25% of patients. Arterial hypotension is related to the extent of the primary myocardial injury,[23] and sometimes to regional ischaemia–reperfusion.[24] Multifocal myocardial injuries cause ventricular dysrhythmias through re-entry mechanisms.[25] Hypotension and dysrhythmias occur during the first two post-traumatic days, especially during general anaesthesia for emergency surgery.[26] The long-term prognosis of myocardial contusion is usually good.[27]

Blunt rupture of the thoracic aorta.   Injury of the aorta is uncommon because aortic disruption is rapidly fatal prior to hospitalization.[28] Injury usually involves the aortic isthmus (90%) at the junction of the mobile and fixed parts of the vessel.[29,30] Survival of the patient after admission depends on the development of a haematoma at the injury site, which is maintained by the intact adventitia. Associated injuries are observed in 95% of these patients, with 10% having a fracture of at least one thoracic vertebra. Evidence suggests that delayed surgical repair will be of benefit in patients who have multiple associated injuries, such as brain injury, lung contusion, or myocardial contusion.[31]

Oesophageal trauma

Blunt oesophageal injury is uncommon. However, sudden compression of the upper abdomen may lead to a burst defect of the lower oesophagus. The development of mediastinitis or pleural empyema may lead to the (delayed) diagnosis of oesophageal rupture.

Primary Assessment and Diagnostic Strategy

Significant chest trauma warrants urgent admission to hospital. Direct patient evaluation is mandatory, including clinical examination, cervical spine, chest and pelvic X-rays, multipurpose ultrasonography, ECG recording, and blood sampling for laboratory investigations. This assessment allows a rapid estimate of overall trauma severity, a rapid diagnosis of all relevant lesions, and treatment prioritization.[32] It is important not to omit *any* of these examinations in patients with severe chest trauma (Fig. 6.2).[33]

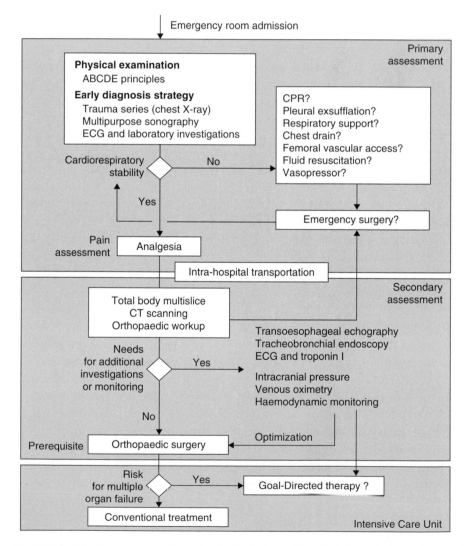

Figure 6.2 Stepwise assessment and diagnosis strategy of the blunt chest trauma patient: upper part, primary assessment, and early resuscitation procedures; middle part, secondary assessment, exhaustive diagnosis, and surgery prerequisites; lower part, final assessment, and prevention of post-traumatic mutiple organ failure.

Physical examination

Clinical examination is central to the detection of cardiorespiratory failure and abnormal neurological status.

A complete primary survey can be challenging in the emergency room. It must be performed in such a manner as to include a quick physical examination and integrate resuscitation procedures. Interventions are based upon clinical status, following the classical ABCDE principles of resuscitation:[34]

A for *airway management* and cervical spine control. A normal voice usually indicates patent airway.

B for *breathing* and ventilation. Anterior and posterior aspects of the thorax are inspected to note any bruises, ecchymoses, subcutaneous emphysema, and other skin marks. Movements of chest and abdomen, and the use of accessory muscles during respiration, may help in assessing lung function. Pulse oximetry is routinely used in all patients to monitor oxygen saturation. However, it may become ineffective if peripheral circulation is impaired, but will often improve when the patient is warmed.[35]

C for *circulation* with haemorrhage control. The expected blood loss may be estimated from the extent of the injuries. Bradycardia associated with arterial hypotension may suggest impairment of cardiovascular homeostatic mechanisms due to the sympatholytic phase of haemorrhagic shock, spinal cord injury, and pharmacological interaction. Distended neck veins may not be apparent in cardiac tamponade or right ventricular failure.

D for *dysfunction* of the central nervous system (CNS). CNS function is assessed by the examination of the pupils, the Glasgow Coma Scale, and the ASIA/IMSOP score for spinal cord injury.[36]

E for full *exposure* of the patient, followed by covering the patient with a warming blanket.

The secondary survey consists of a detailed physical examination while cardiorespiratory function and neurological status are regularly re-evaluated. Allergies (and asthma), Medication, Past medical history (especially cardiorespiratory diseases), Last meal, and Events leading to the injury should be obtained from the patient or relatives (**AMPLE**).[34]

Standard X-rays

A trauma series of X-rays should be obtained in the emergency room to rapidly screen out life-threatening injuries.[34]

The cross table lateral view of the cervical spine has a low ability to identify spinal injury and is usually limited to the upper part of the cervical spine.[37] Nevertheless, a careful examination of the lateral cervical spine X-ray may allow early detection of other serious injuries, which may interfere with respiratory function: for example, fracture of the mandible, airway obstruction from soft tissue swelling or debris, laryngotracheal injuries, endotracheal tube malposition, and even pneumocephalus.[38] Similarly, plain anterior–posterior pelvic radiography is recommended in deceleration or crush injury, and in all multiple injured patients,[39] particularly if there is altered consciousness or neurological impairment.[40] In chest trauma patients, the suprapelvic film should be performed before the patient is sat up for a chest X-ray (CXR).

The CXR is commonly the primary imaging method used for the trauma patient in the emergency room.[2] However, significant numbers of serious chest injuries are missed. The sensitivity for the detection of thoracic injuries depends on patient position: 58% for supine CXR versus 79% for standing CXR. Rib fractures are more frequently detected by CXR than by CT scan.[41] However, CT scan is more likely to identify occult pneumothorax (57% of patients)[42,43] and this will require treatment in 43% of patients.[43] Similarly, the incidence of lung contusion is underestimated by CXR as compared with CT scan (23% versus 40%).[44] Thus, a CXR cannot be used as the sole test for diagnosing or excluding mediastinal injury, particularly aortic disruption.

Mediastinal width depends on patient position and respiratory cycle.[45] The vast majority of patients with an aortic injury have an abnormal initial CXR, with widened mediastinum (85%) and an indistinct aortic knob.[30] A widened mediastinum is highly suggestive of aortic damage or myocardial contusion, whereas high rib and sternal fractures do not have the same predictive value.[46,47]

Sonographic assessment

Ultrasonography, even by a non-radiologist member of the trauma team, can be an important tool in the initial assessment of trauma patients. Ultrasound imaging frequently contributes to the diagnosis of life-threatening injuries by improving the diagnostic value of CXR, and facilitating haemodynamic assessment (Fig. 6.3). The value of hand-held ultrasound devices used for the care of cardiac or trauma patients has not been completely evaluated.[48]

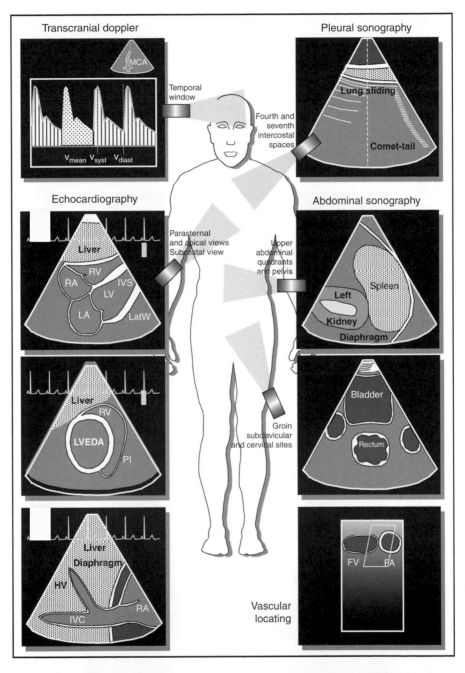

Figure 6.3 Multiple use of ultrasonography during the primary assessment of the blunt chest trauma patient. FA: femoral artery; FV: femoral vein; HV: hepatic vein; IVC: inferior vena cava; IVS: interventricular septum; LA: left atrium; LatW: lateral wall of LV; LVEDA: LV end-diastolic cross sectional area; MCA: mean cerebral artery, RA: right atrium; RV: right ventricle; v_{syst}, v_{mean} and v_{diast}, MCA velocities.

Pleural sonography

The radiological features of pneumothorax may be quite subtle in antero-posterior supine CXR films. Sonography defines a 'lung point', when the fleeting appearance of a lung pattern in the critically ill patient (lung sliding and/or pathological comet-tail artefacts) is replaced by a pneumothorax pattern (absence of lung sliding and exclusive horizontal lines) in a definite location of the chest wall.[49] This ultrasound sign has an overall sensitivity of 66% (75% in radio-occult pneumothorax) and a 100% specificity, and is especially useful following chest trauma (Fig. 6.4).[50]

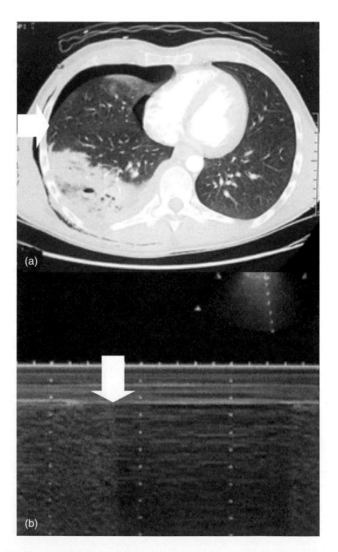

Figure 6.4 Anterior pneumothorax following a blunt chest trauma: (a) CT scanning showing the pneumothorax and a posterior lung contusion; (b) anterior M-mode pleural ultrasonography demonstrating a brutal transition (arrow: 'lung point') between parenchyma on the left and pneumothorax on the right.

Examination of the pleural cavity is performed in both right and left anterolateral aspects of the fourth and seventh intercostal spaces. Ultrasonography is an accurate screening tool for haemothorax with high reported sensitivity (67–100%) and specificity (>99%).[51] Estimation of the volume of haemothorax is performed in the posterior aspect of the right and left ninth intercostal spaces (Fig. 6.5). Formulas to calculate the volume of effusion have not been found to be useful in an emergency setting.[52]

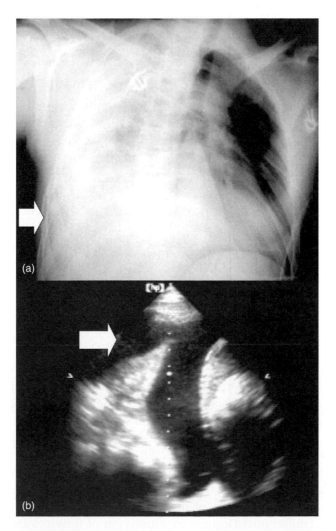

Figure 6.5 Massive haemothorax following blunt chest trauma. (a) CXR showing the right opacity and the mediastinal shift to the left; (b) posterior bidimensional pleural ultrasonography showing the haemothorax (arrow) surrounding the collapsed lung with the diaphragm and the abdominal cavity on the right.

Abdominal sonography

The abdominal examination should include visualization of Morrison's pouch (perihepatic), the perisplenic region and the pelvis before bladder catheter insertion. The presence of parenchymal abnormalities is not the main focus of the examination.[53] The presence or absence of fluid in any of these regions is noted (FAST test; Focused Assessment with Sonography for Trauma).[54] A simple scoring system may be used to semi-quantify the volume of haemoperitoneum.[55] If adequately performed, ultrasonography can detect <50 ml of fluid. The overall sensitivity of abdominal ultrasonography for haemoperitoneum is >98% (specificity >99%) compared with CT scanning, peritoneal lavage, and laparotomy.[56]

Echocardiography

Short-axis plane examination of the left ventricle (LV) at the level of the apex, papillary muscles, and mitral valve is not easy to perform using the parasternal transducer position due to chest pain, subcutaneous emphysema, drain insertion, or bandages.[57,58] The subcostal transducer position is therefore preferred, and may be more useful in these patients even if a perfect short-axis plane is rarely obtained.[59] A LV end-diastolic area below $10\,\text{cm}^2/\text{m}^2$ and a virtual LV end-systolic area index indicate an inadequate LV filling as a result of hypovolaemia or excessive intrathoracic pressure.[60] A long axis plane of the inferior vena cava contributes to the diagnosis of hypovolaemia because its diameter at end-expiration and end-diastole correlates with right atrial pressure in the mechanically ventilated patient. A marked cyclic change of the inferior vena cava diameter during spontaneous ventilation indicates hypovolaemia.[61] Diagnosis of significant pericardial effusion is made by identifying an echo-free space which persists throughout the cardiac cycle. The echo-free space will be between the posterior epicardium initially, followed by the anterior pericardium and the ventricular free wall. The volume of a possible pericardial effusion (echo-free space) can be roughly characterized. Diastolic collapse of the right ventricle and right atrium are sensitive indicators of cardiac tamponade in a similar fashion to pulsus paradoxus in hypovolaemic patients.[62] The echocardiographic criteria used to confirm significant myocardial contusion are pericardial effusion, regional wall motion abnormality, or acute valvular dysfunction (Fig. 6.6).[63]

Transcranial Doppler

The estimation of cerebral perfusion pressure using transcranial Doppler and arterial pressure may be useful in both chest and head-injured patients when invasive measurement of intracranial pressure is neither practical nor safe.[64] Transcranial Doppler measurement of flow-velocity in the M1 portion of the middle cerebral artery throughout the arterial pressure cycle allows estimation of cerebral perfusion pressure.[65] A cerebral perfusion

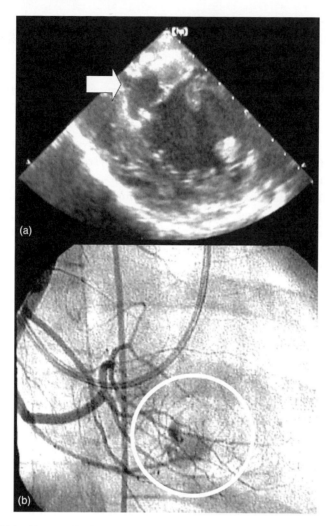

Figure 6.6 Major blunt cardiac injury following blunt chest trauma. (a) Echographic view of a pseudoaneurysm of the LV diaphragmatic wall (arrow). (b) Rupture of a distal branch of a dominant right coronary in the pseudoaneurysm (circle).

pressure ≥ 70 mmHg should be a resuscitation endpoint in brain injured patients with or without chest trauma.[66]

Ultrasound-guided vascular access

Ultrasound guided venous access may improve success rates.[67] This technique may be particularly useful in patients with blunt chest trauma.

ECG recording and cardiac markers assays

All patients should have blood taken for serum troponin concentration and a 12-lead ECG performed on admission. Troponin concentration and

ECG are repeated between 6 and 12 h after admission minimally. Thereafter, troponin concentration and ECG are repeated as clinically indicated.

ECG recording

ECG is neither sensitive nor specific for the diagnosis of blunt cardiac injury but it is the best screening test available in the emergency room.[2] A meta-analysis has demonstrated that an abnormal ECG recording during the primary assessment correlates with severe cardiovascular complications, especially arterial hypotension and ventricular dysrhythmias.[68] The criteria used in making the diagnosis of myocardial contusion was significant of ECG changes after admission and during the period of observation, whatever the circulating troponin concentration.[63] The ECG criteria were defined as conduction abnormality, bundle branch block pattern, prolonged QT-interval, Q-wave formation, ST-segment depression or elevation >1 mm, flat or inverted T-waves or both in two or more leads, and irregular rhythm such as ventricular dysrhythmias, supraventricular tachycardia, atrial fibrillation or flutter, junctional tachycardia and sinus bradycardia.

Determination of troponin concentration

The lack of specificity of the creatine kinase (CK) muscle band (MB)-isoform now explains the low diagnostic value of this marker in patients suffering peripheral muscle injuries.[2] Furthermore, the inability of an elevated CK-MB to be of prognostic value in a chest injured patient has been demonstrated.[69,70] The cardiac isoform of troponin-I (TnI) is never present in skeletal muscle. TnI concentration is a specific indicator of myocardial injury following blunt trauma, but does not appear to have, by itself, a predictive value for the subsequent development of cardiovascular complications.[2] However, a normal ECG recording with absence of TnI release at admission and 8 h later excludes a diagnosis of significant blunt cardiac injury.[71] In our department, a plasma level of cardiac TnI >0.4 μg/l corresponds to a significant myocardial injury. In non-selected trauma patients, three TnI release profiles have been identified:

- A very transient (≤12 h) and limited release (peak TnI <2 μg/l).

- A transient (≤36 h) and significant release (peak TnI ≥2 μg/l).

- A sustained (>36 h) and significant release (peak TnI >2 μg/l).

Whatever the results of the ECG, myocardial injury associated with a recent blunt trauma without any evidence of pre-existing coronary artery disease is considered as an indication for urgent coronary angiography.[72] A sustained and significant release of TnI occurs in 8% of patients and corresponds to coronary artery injury in 41% of these cases.

Secondary Assessment and Surgery Prerequisites

With regard to the chest component of multiple trauma, three injuries require immediate intervention before any intra-hospital transport:

- Major pleural or intrabronchial bleeding following thoracic organ or blood vessel damage.

- Cardiac tamponade.

- Proximal tracheal or bronchial rupture.

In the absence of emergency surgery, the use of whole body, multislice CT becomes a major diagnostic tool. It has been recommended that scanners be installed adjacent to the emergency room to reduce the complications associated with intra-hospital transportation (Fig. 6.2).[73,74]

Whole-body CT scanning

CT scanning is recommended in all patients with major chest trauma whatever the results of initial chest radiograph.[75] The use of CT scanning rather than CXR alone may result in changes in patient management in 41% of the patients.[76]

Lung contusion

The primary CXR usually underestimates the size of lung contusion, which may become evident after 24–48 h. CT scanning accurately identifies the presence and quantifies the size of lung contusion.[8] The need for ventilatory support has been predicted by repeated CXR and arterial blood-gas analysis,[12] or by the percentage of airspace consolidation at the visual analysis of CT scanning.[8] The extent of the contusion volume measured using three-dimensional reconstruction allows for accurate estimation for subsequent development of acute respiratory distress syndrome (ARDS).[77] Patients with more than 20% contusion volume can be predicted to develop ARDS with 90% specificity. Improved contrast bolus imaging, thinner slices, and isotropic voxels permit identification of major organ system disruption and subtle injuries, such as bronchial rupture.[78] The optimal amount of contrast material for single bolus administration in emergency CT examination of the chest and abdomen has to be determined precisely.[79]

Blunt aortic injury

CT scanning has been shown to be a valuable screening test in the diagnosis of blunt aortic injury and mediastinal abnormalities.[2] Contrast-enhanced helical CT has similar diagnostic accuracy to aortography for the identification of significant (surgical) aortic injury.[80] Transoesophageal echocardiography, in experienced hands, is sensitive in detecting intimal or medial lesions of the thoracic aorta and aids the diagnosis of associated cardiac injuries.[81] However, the clinical implications of limited aortic injuries diagnosed by this technique have yet to be fully determined.[82]

Spinal injury

The sensitivity of reformatted helical CT scanning as a screening test for spine fractures is 97% for thoracic injury and 95% for lumbar injury compared with 62% and 86% for conventional radiographs.[83] It has been suggested that CT scanning should replace plain radiographs in high-risk trauma patients.[84]

Associated abdominal injury

CT scanning can be used in patients with stable cardiorespiratory status and positive abdominal ultrasonography during the primary assessment to evaluate whether solid organ injury may be treated conservatively. Moreover free fluid without evidence of organ injury suggests peritoneal diffusion from a retroperitoneal haematoma, or from bowel, mesenteric or bladder injury.[53] Free air, bowel wall thickening, mesenteric infiltration, intravenous contrast media extravasation with or without free fluid are common in bowel or mesenteric injury.[85]

Secondary surgery

The optimal treatment of major fractures in patients with blunt multiple injuries, including chest trauma, is still controversial. A retrospective analysis of 2805 patients in 1994 noted a trend towards higher mortality in the subgroup of patients with femoral shaft fracture, repaired within 1 day, as well as those patients whose surgery was delayed more than 4 days.[86] In patients with severe chest trauma, a higher incidence of post-traumatic ARDS (33% versus 7.7%) and mortality (21% versus 4%) has been noted when easily intramedullary nailing was done in patients who had concomitant chest injuries.[87] In contrast, other authors have shown that early osteosynthesis of femoral shaft fracture decreases the incidence of pulmonary complications in non-selected patients[88] and reduces the incidence of ARDS in chest trauma patients.[89] The incidence of post-operative pulmonary complications depends on the severity of lung contusion,[89] the experience of the trauma team in the management of multiply injured patients,[90] and the presence of several prerequisites before performing early osteosynthesis in polytraumatized patients:[91,92]

multimodal brain monitoring in head-injured patients with the absence of uncontrolled increase in intracranial pressure, absence of hypothermia ($\geq35°C$), absence of clotting problems (prothrombin time <16 s, or $>50\%$: fibrinogen >1 g/l; platelets $>75-100 \times 10^9$/l), stable arterial pressure without recent changes in cardiovascular resuscitation, blood lactate <2.5 mmol/l,[93] and finally a PaO_2/FIO_2 ratio >280 without intra-bronchial bleeding or oedema formation with continuous assessment of pleural drainage. In these circumstances, early temporary stabilization using external fixation reduces the inflammatory syndrome[94] and decreases the incidence of multiple organ failure.[95]

Therapeutic Strategy

Cardiopulmonary resuscitation

Airway obstruction, tension pneumothorax, massive haemothorax, flail chest, extensive lung contusion, and cardiac tamponade can all precipitate cardiac arrest as a result of hypoxaemia and/or exsanguination. Specific medical or surgical treatment is needed to prevent this. Cardiopulmonary resuscitation may be difficult in patients with multiple rib fractures. Emergency thoracotomy enables internal cardiac massage and clamping of the aorta which contributes to the restoration of cerebral and coronary perfusion pressures while reducing the rate of a possible extrathoracic bleed. Emergency thoracotomy should be performed in an operating room by a trained surgeon. The vast majority of salvage thoracotomies for blunt trauma are unsuccessful because the injuries discovered are irreparable. Absence of signs of life at the scene of injury and prolonged cardiopulmonary resuscitation represent contraindications to this futile procedure.[96]

Analgesia

Pain relief is a major component of medical management because deep inspiration and coughing are extremely painful. The needs for analgesia have to be assessed at rest and during effective respiratory care. Pain (visual analogic scale) and respiratory assessments (respiratory rate, effort, and symmetry) should be simultaneous.

Systemic analgesia

Analgesics should be chosen that act on all components of pain.[97] Paracetamol and/or nefopam, in association with a non-steroidal anti-inflammatory drug such as ibuprofen and with intravenous morphine may be effective.

Regional analgesia
Intercostal nerve block using a catheter may be used in patients with coagulopathy or spinal cord injury but the pain relief will be limited to three to five homolateral intercostal spaces.[98] The efficacy of pleural analgesia is short-lived, due to anaesthetic resorption by inflamed pleura. Pleural injection of local anaesthetic does not reduce the morphine requirements during the first post-traumatic day and is less effective than epidural analgesia.[99,100]

Pulmonary morbidity and overall mortality following thoracic trauma is increased in elderly patients.[101] Peridural analgesia may improve pulmonary function and modify the immune response.[102] Sympathetic activity to the lower part of the body is only partially blocked by low dose local anaesthetic infusions, thus preventing the deleterious effect on haemodynamic stability.[103,104] As access to the thoracic epidural space is not always easy, it is noteworthy that epidural infusion of opiates alone, whatever the level of injection, improves tolerance to respiratory physiotherapy and of non-invasive ventilation.[105] Epidural infusion of morphine or fentanyl at the lumbar level is more effective than an intravenous infusion of morphine or fentanyl.[106,107]

Paravertebral block is an alternative to epidural block in a unilateral chest trauma patient with brain or spinal cord injury, coagulopathy or ventilatory support. The injection of local anaesthetic adjacent to the thoracic vertebra in close proximity to the spinal nerve as it emerges from the intervertebral foramina, results in ipsilateral somatic and sympathetic nerve blockade in multiple contiguous thoracic dermatomes above and below the site of injection.[108] A single injection of 25 ml of local anaesthetic results in prolonged pain relief.[109] After a bolus dose, a continuous paravertebral infusion may be used.[108]

Pain management
A step-by-step approach to analgesia is required in chest trauma patients.[110] All non-intubated patients with blunt chest trauma should be given supplementary oxygen and multiple-drug systemic analgesia. Injection of local anaesthetic in the pleural cavity in addition to chest wall infiltration may be effective for early chest drain insertion. If residual pain is excessive, or if the respiratory care is inadequate because of pain, continuous epidural anaesthesia or thoracic paravertebral block should be instituted before anti-deep venous thrombosis prophylaxis. Regional anaesthesia permits the effective application of pressure support ventilation through a face mask. If tracheal intubation and mechanical ventilation become indicated during the evolution, regional anaesthesia decreases the needs for concomitant sedation.

Respiratory care

Intercostal drainage

A chest drain is necessary in case of complete pneumothorax, respiratory failure or partial pneumothorax in haemodynamically unstable patients, before transport, and if intermittent positive pressure ventilation is needed. The significance of a partial pneumothorax is defined by its size on thoracic CT scanning (thickness >5 mm and height >80 mm);[111] thoracic ultrasonography is probably equivalent to CT for this assessment. A chest drain should be inserted before general anaesthesia for emergency surgery whatever the size of pneumothorax.[112]

A chest drain is needed for decompressing the chest cavity in case of massive haemothorax. Sudden decompression may lead to haemodynamic decompensation if the source of bleeding is not controlled. Intermittent suction may be employed, with re-infusion of collected blood before therapeutic thoracotomy.[113] A chest drain should be inserted when the sonographic width of the pleural effusion is >15 mm, to prevent lung collapse and subsequent infection and pleural empyema.[114]

Mechanical ventilation

The prognosis of organ failure, treatment time, and mortality is unaffected in patients with severe thoracic trauma, if these patients do not have respiratory insufficiency prior to hospital admission.[115] Tracheal intubation and mechanical ventilation is indicated when three of the five following criteria are present:

- Respiratory rate >25 bpm.
- PaO_2 <8 kPa (60 mmHg) with FIO_2 >0.6 or $PaCO_2$ >7.5 kPa (55 mmHg).
- Systolic arterial pressure <100 mmHg despite fluid resuscitation.
- Heart rate >100 bpm.
- Severe head (Glasgow Coma Scale <9) or abdominal injury.[13,116]

A low respiratory rate may improve the coronary artery perfusion in haemodynamically unstable trauma patients.[117] Fluid requirements are significantly higher in intubated chest trauma patients.[115] In the absence of altered consciousness or shock, the requirement for tracheal intubation needs to be assessed after adequate analgesia, chest drain insertion, and non-invasive ventilation.[118] Pressure support is usually employed during spontaneous ventilation with a low level of positive end-expiratory pressure and an FIO_2 of 0.5. Non-invasive ventilation as compared with tracheal intubation reduces the incidence of pneumopathy (44% versus 6%) and overall mortality (27% versus 0%) of patients with blunt chest trauma.[13] The reasons for failure of non-invasive ventilation are inadequate respiratory care, underestimation of injuries, associated injuries, and pulmonary infection.

Cardiovascular care

Haemodynamic stability

Arterial hypotension is usually related to hypovolaemia in trauma patients but haemodynamic instability may be exacerbated by pleural effusion, myocardial dysfunction, or loss of vascular tone due to spinal cord injury or early systemic inflammatory response syndrome.[119] Aggressive fluid resuscitation of an hypotensive patient may result in rebleeding and subsequent increase in mortality.[120] A limited, or controlled, or delayed resuscitation of shock patients has been suggested to limit the deleterious consequences of excessive fluid infusion.[121] Permissive arterial hypotension (systolic arterial pressure of about 85–90 mmHg) has been suggested for bleeding patients following surgical haemostasis in the absence of CNS injury (see Recent Advances in Anaesthesia and Analgesic No 21). Optimized arterial pressure (systolic arterial pressure about 110–120 mmHg) is the goal for the remaining patients, and arterial hypertension should be avoided, especially when an aortic injury is suspected.[122]

An increase in pulmonary extravascular water has been reported following crystalloid resuscitation in chest trauma patients without impairment of gas exchange or increase in mortality.[123–125] However, excessive fluid resuscitation with crystalloid is an independent factor for acute lung injury in trauma patients.[11] A clear advantage of colloid solution resuscitation has not been demonstrated.[126] Vasopressor infusion is frequently used to reach the targeted arterial pressure when the volume of fluids replaced corresponds to the estimated blood loss.[34] Blood products are transfused to maintain haemoglobin $\geqslant 7$ g/dl, prothrombin time $\leqslant 16$ s ($\geqslant 40\%$), fibrinogen $\geqslant 1$ g/l, and platelets count $\geqslant 75 \times 10^9$/l.[127] The femoral approach will rapidly obtain effective and safe vascular access in patients with chest trauma.[128,129]

Post-traumatic goal-directed therapy

Multiple organ failure can be predicted as early as 12 h following injury by using a checklist to specific criteria: severe torso trauma ($\geqslant 2$ abdominal organs, $\geqslant 3$ rib fractures, major vascular injury, complex pelvic fracture, and/or 2 long bone fractures), anticipated need for $\geqslant 6$ units of packed red cells transfusion, and early base-deficit $\geqslant 6$ mmol/l (Fig. 6.2).[130,131] To prevent multiple organ failure, a resuscitation strategy based on a standardized process using oxygen delivery as an endpoint has been evaluated in prospective trials of trauma patient outcome.[132] Fluid and blood are used predominantly with or without inotropes. However, the routine insertion of a pulmonary artery catheter is controversial, and 'supranormal' resuscitation can cause abdominal compartment syndrome and pulmonary oedema which are obviously deleterious following a blunt chest trauma.[132] Early and less invasive strategies should be developed following trauma to drive the patient towards an optimal cardiorespiratory status.[133,134] A standard protocol seems to be more important than the specific endpoints.[132]

Prevention of deep venous thrombosis

Chest trauma is a major cause of deep venous thrombosis.[135] Normovolaemic haemodilution and early intermittent pneumatic compression are indicated. The use of low molecular weight heparin is more effective than unfractionated heparin.[136,137] In the absence of early and adequate prophylaxis prior to the second post-traumatic day, Doppler sonography should be employed to identify deep venous thrombosis, but conventional phlebography remains the 'gold standard' reference in trauma patients.[138]

Conclusion

Blunt chest trauma remains a clinical challenge because life-threatening chest lesions are frequently associated with extrathoracic injuries, and contribute to a severe and sometimes delayed cardiorespiratory failure. The use of new imaging technology with standardized procedures gives a great opportunity for early and meticulous assessment in trauma patients. Adequate and specific stepwise therapeutic strategies are based on multimodal analgesia and aggressive cardiorespiratory resuscitation using noninvasive ventilatory support and haemodynamic optimization.

Acknowledgements

The authors gratefully acknowledge the help of Tohme Wissam in preparing this manuscript.

References

1. LoCicero III J, Mattox KL. Epidemiology of chest trauma. Surg Clin North Am 1989; 69: 15–19.
2. Greenberg MD, Rosen CL. Evaluation of the patient with blunt chest trauma: an evidence based approach. Emerg Med Clin North Am 1999; 17: 41–62.
3. Moore EE, Cogbill TH, Malangoni MA *et al*. Organ injury scaling. Surg Clin North Am 1995; 75: 293–303.

4. Pate JW. Chest wall injuries. Surg Clin North Am 1989; 69: 59–70.
5. Chiu WC, D'Amelio LF, Hammond JS. Sternal fractures in blunt chest trauma: a practical algorithm for management. Am J Emerg Med 1997; 15: 252–255.
6. Stephens NG, Morgan AS, Corvo P, Bernstein BA. Significance of scapular fracture in the blunt-trauma patient. Ann Emerg Med 1995; 26: 439–442.
7. Gelman R, Mirvis SE, Gens D. Diaphragmatic rupture due to blunt trauma: sensitivity of plain chest radiographs. Am J Roentgenol 1991; 156: 51–57.
8. Wagner RB, Jamieson PM. Pulmonary contusion. Evaluation and classification by computed tomography. Surg Clin North Am 1989; 69: 31–40.
9. Hellinger A, Konerding MA, Malkusch W et al. Does lung contusion affect both the traumatized and the noninjured lung parenchyma? A morphological and morphometric study in the pig. J Trauma 1995; 39: 712–719.
10. Richardson JD, Woods D, Johanson Jr WG, Trinkle JK. Lung bacterial clearance following pulmonary contusion. Surgery 1979; 86: 730–735.
11. Eberhard LW, Morabito DJ, Matthay MA et al. Initial severity of metabolic acidosis predicts the development of acute lung injury in severely traumatized patients. Crit Care Med 2000; 28: 125–131.
12. Tyburski JG, Collinge JD, Wilson RF, Eachempati SR. Pulmonary contusions: quantifying the lesions on chest X-ray films and the factors affecting prognosis. J Trauma 1999; 46: 833–838.
13. Richardson JD, Adams L, Flint LM. Selective management of flail chest and pulmonary contusion. Ann Surg 1982; 196: 481–487.
14. Van Eeden SF, Klopper JF, Alheit B, Bardin PG. Ventilation–perfusion imaging in evaluating regional lung function in nonpenetrating injury to the chest. Chest 1989; 95: 632–638.
15. Kishikawa M, Yoshioka T, Shimazu T, Sugimoto H, Sugimoto T. Pulmonary contusion causes long-term respiratory dysfunction with decreased functional residual capacity. J Trauma 1991; 31: 1203–1208.
16. Shorr RM, Crittenden M, Indeck M, Hartunian SL, Rodriguez A. Blunt thoracic trauma. Analysis of 515 patients. Ann Surg 1987; 206: 200–205.
17. Pate JW. Tracheobronchial and esophageal injuries. Surg Clin North Am 1989; 69: 111–123.
18. Pretre R, Chilcott M. Blunt trauma to the heart and great vessels. New Engl J Med 1997; 336: 626–632.
19. Orliaguet G, Ferjani M, Riou B. The heart in blunt trauma. Anesthesiology 2001; 95: 544–548.
20. Hackel DB, Ratliff NB, Mikat E. The heart in shock. Circ Res 1974; 35: 805–811.
21. Catoire P, Orliaguet G, Liu N et al. Systematic transesophageal echocardiography for detection of mediastinal lesions in patients with multiple injuries. J Trauma 1995; 38: 96–102.
22. Edouard AR, Benoist JF, Cosson C, Mimoz O, Legrand A, Samii K. Circulating cardiac troponin I in trauma patients without cardiac contusion. Intens Care Med 1998; 24: 569–573.
23. Utley JR, Doty DB, Collins JC, Spaw EA, Wachtel C, Todd EP. Cardiac output, coronary flow, ventricular fibrillation and survival following varying degrees of myocardial contusion. J Surg Res 1976; 20: 539–543.
24. Liedtke AJ, Allen RP, Nellis SH. Effects of blunt cardiac trauma on coronary vasomotion, perfusion, myocardial mechanics, and metabolism. J Trauma 1980; 20: 777–785.

25. Robert E, de La Coussaye JE, Aya AG *et al*. Mechanisms of ventricular arrhythmias induced by myocardial contusion: a high-resolution mapping study in left ventricular rabbit heart. Anesthesiology 2000; 92: 1132–1143.
26. Devitt JH, McLean RF, McLellan BA. Perioperative cardiovascular complications associated with blunt thoracic trauma. Can J Anaesth 1993; 40: 197–200.
27. Lindstaedt M, Germing A, Lawo T *et al*. Acute and long-term clinical significance of myocardial contusion following blunt thoracic trauma: results of a prospective study. J Trauma 2002; 52: 479–485.
28. Feczko JD, Lynch L, Pless JE, Clark MA, McClain J, Hawley DA. An autopsy case review of 142 nonpenetrating (blunt) injuries of the aorta. J Trauma 1992; 33: 846–849.
29. Cowley RA, Turney SZ, Hankins JR, Rodriguez A, Attar S, Shankar BS. Rupture of thoracic aorta caused by blunt trauma. A fifteen-year experience. J Thorac Cardiovasc Surg 1990; 100: 652–660.
30. Fabian TC, Richardson JD, Croce MA *et al*. Prospective study of blunt aortic injury: Multicenter Trial of the American Association for the Surgery of Trauma. J Trauma 1997; 42: 374–380.
31. Pate JW, Fabian TC, Walker WA. Acute traumatic rupture of the aortic isthmus: repair with cardiopulmonary bypass. Ann Thorac Surg 1995; 59: 90–98.
32. Ruchholtz S, Zintl B, Nast-Kolb D *et al*. Improvement in the therapy of multiply injured patients by introduction of clinical management guidelines. Injury 1998; 29: 115–129.
33. Peytel E, Menegaux F, Cluzel P, Langeron O, Coriat P, Riou B. Initial imaging assessment of severe blunt trauma. Intens Care Med 2001; 27: 1756–1761.
34. Leenen L, Goris R. Standard diagnostic workup of the severely traumatized patient. In: Goris R, Trentz O (eds). The Integrated Approach to Trauma Patient Care. The First 24 Hours. Berlin/Heidelberg: Springer Verlag, 1995; 106–113.
35. Kober A, Scheck T, Lieba F *et al*. The influence of active warming on signal quality of pulse oximetry in prehospital trauma care. Anesth Analg 2002; 95: 961–966.
36. ASIA/IMSOP. International standards for neurological and functional classification of spinal cord injury, Revised 1998. Chicago: American Spinal Injury Association; 1998.
37. Shaffer MA, Doris PE. Limitation of the cross table lateral view in detecting cervical spine injuries: a retrospective analysis. Ann Emerg Med 1981; 10: 508–513.
38. Perry JR, Stern EJ, Mann FA, Baxter AB. Lateral radiography of the cervical spine in the trauma patient: looking beyond the spine. Am J Roentgenol 2001; 176: 381–386.
39. Bucholz RW. Injuries of the pelvis and hip. Emerg Med Clin North Am 1984; 2: 331–346.
40. Civil ID, Ross SE, Botehlo G, Schwab CW. Routine pelvic radiography in severe blunt trauma: is it necessary? Ann Emerg Med 1988; 17: 488–490.
41. Smejkal R, O'Malley KF, David E, Cernaianu AC, Ross SE. Routine initial computed tomography of the chest in blunt torso trauma. Chest 1991; 100: 667–669.
42. Bridges KG, Welch G, Silver M, Schinco MA, Esposito B. CT detection of occult pneumothorax in multiple trauma patients. J Emerg Med 1993; 11: 179–186.
43. Wolfman NT, Gilpin JW, Bechtold RE, Meredith JW, Ditesheim JA. Occult pneumothorax in patients with abdominal trauma: CT studies. J Comput Assist Tomogr 1993; 17: 56–59.

44. Karaaslan T, Meuli R, Androux R, Duvoisin B, Hessler C, Schnyder P. Traumatic chest lesions in patients with severe head trauma: a comparative study with computed tomography and conventional chest roentgenograms. J Trauma 1995; 39: 1081–1086.

45. Lee Jr FT, Katzberg RW, Gutierrez OH et al. Reevaluation of plain radiographic findings in the diagnosis of aortic rupture: the role of inspiration and positioning on mediastinal width. J Emerg Med 1993; 11: 289–296.

46. Hills MW, Delprado AM, Deane SA. Sternal fractures: associated injuries and management. J Trauma 1993; 35: 55–60.

47. Lee J, Harris Jr JH, Duke Jr JH, Williams JS. Noncorrelation between thoracic skeletal injuries and acute traumatic aortic tear. J Trauma 1997; 43: 400–404.

48. Seward JB, Douglas PS, Erbel R et al. Hand-carried cardiac ultrasound (HCU) device: recommendations regarding new technology. A report from the Echocardiography Task Force on New Technology of the Nomenclature and Standards Committee of the American Society of Echocardiography. J Am Soc Echocardiogr 2002; 15: 369–373.

49. Chan SS. Emergency bedside ultrasound to detect pneumothorax. Acad Emerg Med 2003; 10: 91–94.

50. Lichtenstein D, Meziere G, Biderman P, Gepner A. The 'lung point': an ultrasound sign specific to pneumothorax. Intens Care Med 2000; 26: 1434–1440.

51. Abboud PA, Kendall J. Emergency department ultrasound for haemothorax after blunt traumatic injury. J Emerg Med 2003; 25: 181–184.

52. Beckh S, Bolcskei PL, Lessnau KD. Real-time chest ultrasonography: a comprehensive review for the pulmonologist. Chest 2002; 122: 1759–1773.

53. Fabian TC, Croce MA, Minard G et al. Current issues in trauma. Curr Probl Surg 2002; 39: 1160–1244.

54. Scalea TM, Rodriguez A, Chiu WC et al. Focused Assessment with Sonography for Trauma (FAST): results from an international consensus conference. J Trauma 1999; 46: 466–472.

55. Huang MS, Liu M, Wu JK, Shih HC, Ko TJ, Lee CH. Ultrasonography for the evaluation of haemoperitoneum during resuscitation: a simple scoring system. J Trauma 1994; 36: 173–177.

56. McKenney MG, Martin L, Lentz K et al. 1000 consecutive ultrasounds for blunt abdominal trauma. J Trauma 1996; 40: 607–610; discussion 611–612.

57. Brooks SW, Young JC, Cmolik B et al. The use of transesophageal echocardiography in the evaluation of chest trauma. J Trauma 1992; 32: 761–765.

58. Karalis DG, Victor MF, Davis GA et al. The role of echocardiography in blunt chest trauma: a transthoracic and transesophageal echocardiographic study. J Trauma 1994; 36: 53–58.

59. Seward J, Tajik A, Hagler D, Edwards W. Nomenclature, image orientation and anatomic-echocardiographic correlations with tomographic views. In: Schapira J, Harold J (eds). Two-Dimensional Echocardiography and Cardiac Doppler. Baltimore: Williams and Wilkins; 1990.

60. Vieillard-Baron A, Prin S, Chergui K, Dubourg O, Jardin F. Haemodynamic instability in sepsis: bedside assessment by Doppler echocardiography. Am J Respir Crit Care Med 2003; 168: 1270–1276.

61. Bendjelid K, Romand JA, Walder B, Suter PM, Fournier G. Correlation between measured inferior vena cava diameter and right atrial pressure depends on the

echocardiographic method used in patients who are mechanically ventilated. J Am Soc Echocardiogr 2002; 15: 944–949.

62. Cogswell TL, Bernath GA, Wann LS, Hoffman RG, Brooks HL, Klopfenstein HS. Effects of intravascular volume state on the value of pulsus paradoxus and right ventricular diastolic collapse in predicting cardiac tamponade. Circulation 1985; 72: 1076–1080.

63. Bertinchant JP, Polge A, Mohty D *et al*. Evaluation of incidence, clinical significance, and prognostic value of circulating cardiac troponin I and T elevation in haemodynamically stable patients with suspected myocardial contusion after blunt chest trauma. J Trauma 2000; 48: 924–931.

64. Schmidt B, Czosnyka M, Klingelhofer J. Clinical applications of a non-invasive ICP monitoring method. Eur J Ultrasound 2002; 16: 37–45.

65. Belfort MA, Tooke-Miller C, Allen Jr JC *et al*. Changes in flow velocity, resistance indices, and cerebral perfusion pressure in the maternal middle cerebral artery distribution during normal pregnancy. Acta Obstet Gynecol Scand 2001; 80: 104–112.

66. Rosner MJ, Rosner SD, Johnson AH. Cerebral perfusion pressure: management protocol and clinical results. J Neurosurg 1995; 83: 949–962.

67. Randolph AG, Cook DJ, Gonzales CA, Pribble CG. Ultrasound guidance for placement of central venous catheters: a meta-analysis of the literature. Crit Care Med 1996; 24: 2053–2058.

68. Maenza RL, Seaberg D, D'Amico F. A meta-analysis of blunt cardiac trauma: ending myocardial confusion. Am J Emerg Med 1996; 14: 237–241.

69. Soliman MH, Waxman K. Value of a conventional approach to the diagnosis of traumatic cardiac contusion after chest injury. Crit Care Med 1987; 15: 218–220.

70. Wisner DH, Reed WH, Riddick RS. Suspected myocardial contusion. Triage and indications for monitoring. Ann Surg 1990; 212: 82–86.

71. Velmahos GC, Karaiskakis M, Salim A *et al*. Normal electrocardiography and serum troponin I levels preclude the presence of clinically significant blunt cardiac injury. J Trauma 2003; 54: 45–50.

72. Scanlon PJ, Faxon DP, Audet AM *et al*. ACC/AHA guidelines for coronary angiography: executive summary and recommendations. A report of the American College of Cardiology/American Heart Association Task Force on Practice Guidelines (Committee on Coronary Angiography) developed in collaboration with the Society for Cardiac Angiography and Interventions. Circulation 1999; 99: 2345–2357.

73. Sumann G, Kampfl A, Wenzel V, Schobersberger W. Early intensive care unit intervention for trauma care: what alters the outcome? Curr Opin Crit Care 2002; 8: 587–592.

74. Rivas LA, Fishman JE, Munera F, Bajayo DE. Multislice CT in thoracic trauma. Radiol Clin North Am 2003; 41: 599–616.

75. Exadaktylos AK, Sclabas G, Schmid SW, Schaller B, Zimmermann H. Do we really need routine computed tomographic scanning in the primary evaluation of blunt chest trauma in patients with 'normal' chest radiograph? J Trauma 2001; 51: 1173–1176.

76. Trupka A, Waydhas C, Hallfeldt KK, Nast-Kolb D, Pfeifer KJ, Schweiberer L. Value of thoracic computed tomography in the first assessment of severely injured patients with blunt chest trauma: results of a prospective study. J Trauma 1997; 43: 405–411.

77. Miller PR, Croce MA, Bee TK *et al*. ARDS after pulmonary contusion: accurate measurement of contusion volume identifies high-risk patients. J Trauma 2001; 51: 223–228.
78. Wintermark M, Schnyder P, Wicky S. Blunt traumatic rupture of a mainstem bronchus: spiral CT demonstration of the 'fallen lung' sign. Eur Radiol 2001; 11: 409–411.
79. Rademacher G, Stengel D, Siegmann S, Petersein J, Mutze S. Optimization of contrast agent volume for helical CT in the diagnostic assessment of patients with severe and multiple injuries. J Comput Assist Tomogr 2002; 26: 113–118.
80. Parker MS, Matheson TL, Rao AV *et al*. Making the transition: the role of helical CT in the evaluation of potentially acute thoracic aortic injuries. Am J Roentgenol 2001; 176: 1267–1272.
81. Vignon P, Boncoeur MP, Francois B, Rambaud G, Maubon A, Gastinne H. Comparison of multiplane transesophageal echocardiography and contrast-enhanced helical CT in the diagnosis of blunt traumatic cardiovascular injuries. Anesthesiology 2001; 94: 615–622.
82. Goarin JP, Cluzel P, Gosgnach M, Lamine K, Coriat P, Riou B. Evaluation of transesophageal echocardiography for diagnosis of traumatic aortic injury. Anesthesiology 2000; 93: 1373–1377.
83. Sheridan R, Peralta R, Rhea J, Ptak T, Novelline R. Reformatted visceral protocol helical computed tomographic scanning allows conventional radiographs of the thoracic and lumbar spine to be eliminated in the evaluation of blunt trauma patients. J Trauma 2003; 55: 665–669.
84. Hauser CJ, Visvikis G, Hinrichs C *et al*. Prospective validation of computed tomographic screening of the thoracolumbar spine in trauma. J Trauma 2003; 55: 228–234.
85. Brody JM, Leighton DB, Murphy BL *et al*. CT of blunt trauma bowel and mesenteric injury: typical findings and pitfalls in diagnosis. Radiographics 2000; 20: 1525–1536.
86. Fakhry SM, Rutledge R, Dahners LE, Kessler D. Incidence, management, and outcome of femoral shaft fracture: a statewide population-based analysis of 2805 adult patients in a rural state. J Trauma 1994; 37: 255–260.
87. Pape HC, Auf'm'Kolk M, Paffrath T, Regel G, Sturm JA, Tscherne H. Primary intramedullary femur fixation in multiple trauma patients with associated lung contusion – a cause of posttraumatic ARDS? J Trauma 1993; 34: 540–547.
88. Bone LB, Johnson KD, Weigelt J, Scheinberg R. Early versus delayed stabilization of femoral fractures. A prospective randomized study. J Bone Joint Surg Am 1989; 71: 336–340.
89. Boulanger BR, Stephen D, Brenneman FD. Thoracic trauma and early intramedullary nailing of femur fractures: are we doing harm? J Trauma 1997; 43: 24–28.
90. Smith Jr JS, Martin LF, Young WW, Macioce DP. Do trauma centers improve outcome over non-trauma centers: the evaluation of regional trauma care using discharge abstract data and patient management categories. J Trauma 1990; 30: 1533–1538.
91. Biert J, Goris R. Treatment of extremity injuries in polytraumatized patients: timing of osteosynthesis and other important factors. In: Goris R, Trentz O (eds). The Integrated Approach to Trauma Patient Care. The First 24 Hours. Berlin Heidelberg: Springer Verlag; 1995; 219–232.
92. Tscherne H, Regel G, Pape HC, Pohlemann T, Krettek C. Internal fixation of multiple fractures in patients with polytrauma. Clin Orthop 1998; 62–78.

93. Crowl AC, Young JS, Kahler DM, Claridge JA, Chrzanowski DS, Pomphrey M. Occult hypoperfusion is associated with increased morbidity in patients undergoing early femur fracture fixation. J Trauma 2000; 48: 260–267.

94. Pape HC, Grimme K, Van Griensven M *et al.* Impact of intramedullary instrumentation versus damage control for femoral fractures on immunoinflammatory parameters: prospective randomized analysis by the EPOFF Study Group. J Trauma 2003; 55: 7–13.

95. Pape HC, Hildebrand F, Pertschy S *et al.* Changes in the management of femoral shaft fractures in polytrauma patients: from early total care to damage control orthopedic surgery. J Trauma 2002; 53: 452–461.

96. Mattox KL. Indications for thoracotomy: deciding to operate. Surg Clin North Am 1989; 69: 47–58.

97. Kavanagh BP, Katz J, Sandler AN. Pain control after thoracic surgery. A review of current techniques. Anesthesiology 1994; 81: 737–759.

98. Haenel JB, Moore FA, Moore EE, Sauaia A, Read RA, Burch JM. Extrapleural bupivacaine for amelioration of multiple rib fracture pain. J Trauma 1995; 38: 22–27.

99. Luchette FA, Radafshar SM, Kaiser R, Flynn W, Hassett JM. Prospective evaluation of epidural versus intrapleural catheters for analgesia in chest wall trauma. J Trauma 1994; 36: 865–869.

100. Short K, Scheeres D, Mlakar J, Dean R. Evaluation of intrapleural analgesia in the management of blunt traumatic chest wall pain: a clinical trial. Am Surg 1996; 62: 488–493.

101. Peterson RJ, Tepas III JJ, Edwards FH, Kissoon N, Pieper P, Ceithaml EL. Pediatric and adult thoracic trauma: age-related impact on presentation and outcome. Ann Thorac Surg 1994; 58: 14–18.

102. Moon MR, Luchette FA, Gibson SW *et al.* Prospective, randomized comparison of epidural versus parenteral opioid analgesia in thoracic trauma. Ann Surg 1999; 229: 684–691.

103. Hopf HB, Weissbach B, Peters J. High thoracic segmental epidural anesthesia diminishes sympathetic outflow to the legs, despite restriction of sensory blockade to the upper thorax. Anesthesiology 1990; 73: 882–889.

104. Magnusdottir H, Kirno K, Ricksten SE, Elam M. High thoracic epidural anesthesia does not inhibit sympathetic nerve activity in the lower extremities. Anesthesiology 1999; 91: 1299–1304.

105. Bolliger CT, Van Eeden SF. Treatment of multiple rib fractures. Randomized controlled trial comparing ventilatory with nonventilatory management. Chest 1990; 97: 943–948.

106. Ullman DA, Fortune JB, Greenhouse BB, Wimpy RE, Kennedy TM. The treatment of patients with multiple rib fractures using continuous thoracic epidural narcotic infusion. Reg Anesth 1989; 14: 43–47.

107. Guinard JP, Mavrocordatos P, Chiolero R, Carpenter RL. A randomized comparison of intravenous versus lumbar and thoracic epidural fentanyl for analgesia after thoracotomy. Anesthesiology 1992; 77: 1108–1115.

108. Karmakar MK. Thoracic paravertebral block. Anesthesiology 2001; 95: 771–780.

109. Gilbert J, Hultman J. Thoracic paravertebral block: a method of pain control. Acta Anaesthesiol Scand 1989; 33: 142–145.

110. Frutiger A, Leutenegger A, Ruedi T. Serial rib fractures: a differentiated treatment concept, illustrated by 59 severely injured intensive care patients. Helv Chir Acta 1990; 57: 279–284.

111. Garramone Jr RR, Jacobs LM, Sahdev P. An objective method to measure and manage occult pneumothorax. Surg Gynecol Obstet 1991; 173: 257–261.

112. Enderson BL, Abdalla R, Frame SB, Casey MT, Gould H, Maull KI. Tube thoracostomy for occult pneumothorax: a prospective randomized study of its use. J Trauma 1993; 35: 726–729.

113. Barriot P, Riou B, Viars P. Prehospital autotransfusion in life-threatening haemothorax. Chest 1988; 93: 522–526.

114. Eddy AC, Luna GK, Copass M. Empyema thoracis in patients undergoing emergent closed tube thoracostomy for thoracic trauma. Am J Surg 1989; 157: 494–497.

115. Ruchholtz S, Waydhas C, Ose C, Lewan U, Nast-Kolb D. Prehospital intubation in severe thoracic trauma without respiratory insufficiency: a matched-pair analysis based on the Trauma Registry of the German Trauma Society. J Trauma 2002; 52: 879–886.

116. Barone JE, Pizzi WF, Nealon Jr TF, Richman H. Indications for intubation in blunt chest trauma. J Trauma 1986; 26: 334–338.

117. Pepe PE, Raedler C, Lurie KG, Wigginton JG. Emergency ventilatory management in haemorrhagic states: elemental or detrimental? J Trauma 2003; 54: 1048–1055.

118. Walz M, Mollenhoff G, Muhr G. CPAP-augmented spontaneous respiration in thoracic trauma. An alternative to intubation. Unfallchirurg 1998; 101: 527–536.

119. Smail N, Messiah A, Edouard A et al. Role of systemic inflammatory response syndrome and infection in the occurrence of early multiple organ dysfunction syndrome following severe trauma. Intens Care Med 1995; 21: 813–816.

120. Bickell WH, Wall Jr MJ, Pepe PE et al. Immediate versus delayed fluid resuscitation for hypotensive patients with penetrating torso injuries. N Engl J Med 1994; 331: 1105–1109.

121. Dutton RP, Mackenzie CF, Scalea TM. Hypotensive resuscitation during active haemorrhage: impact on in-hospital mortality. J Trauma 2002; 52: 1141–1146.

122. Dries DJ. Hypotensive resuscitation. Shock 1996; 6: 311–316.

123. Tranbaugh RF, Elings VB, Christensen J, Lewis FR. Determinants of pulmonary interstitial fluid accumulation after trauma. J Trauma 1982; 22: 820–826.

124. Bongard FS, Lewis FR. Crystalloid resuscitation of patients with pulmonary contusion. Am J Surg 1984; 148: 145–151.

125. Johnson JA, Cogbill TH, Winga ER. Determinants of outcome after pulmonary contusion. J Trauma 1986; 26: 695–697.

126. Choi PT, Yip G, Quinonez LG, Cook DJ. Crystalloids vs. colloids in fluid resuscitation: a systematic review. Crit Care Med 1999; 27: 200–210.

127. Drummond JC, Petrovitch CT. The massively bleeding patient. Anesthesiol Clin North Am 2001; 19: 633–649.

128. Mangiante EC, Hoots AV, Fabian TC. The percutaneous common femoral vein catheter for volume replacement in critically injured patients. J Trauma 1988; 28: 1644–1649.

129. Westfall MD, Price KR, Lambert M et al. Intravenous access in the critically ill trauma patient: a multicentered, prospective, randomized trial of saphenous cutdown and percutaneous femoral access. Ann Emerg Med 1994; 23: 541–545.

130. Sauaia A, Moore FA, Moore EE, Norris JM, Lezotte DC, Hamman RF. Multiple organ failure can be predicted as early as 12 hours after injury. J Trauma 1998; 45: 291–301.

131. Sauaia A, Moore FA, Moore EE, Haenel JB, Read RA, Lezotte DC. Early predictors of postinjury multiple organ failure. Arch Surg 1994; 129: 39–45.

132. McKinley BA, Valdivia A, Moore FA. Goal-oriented shock resuscitation for major torso trauma: what are we learning? Curr Opin Crit Care 2003; 9: 292–299.

133. Velmahos GC, Wo CC, Demetriades D, Shoemaker WC. Early continuous noninvasive haemodynamic monitoring after severe blunt trauma. Injury 1999; 30: 209–214.

134. McKinley BA, Kozar RA, Cocanour CS et al. Normal versus supranormal oxygen delivery goals in shock resuscitation: the response is the same. J Trauma 2002; 53: 825–832.

135. Geerts WH, Code KI, Jay RM, Chen E, Szalai JP. A prospective study of venous thromboembolism after major trauma. N Engl J Med 1994; 331: 1601–1606.

136. Geerts WH, Jay RM, Code KI et al. A comparison of low-dose heparin with low-molecular-weight heparin as prophylaxis against venous thromboembolism after major trauma. N Engl J Med 1996; 335: 701–707.

137. Geerts WH, Heit JA, Clagett GP et al. Prevention of venous thromboembolism. Chest 2001; 119: 132S–175S.

138. Spinal Cord Injury Thromboproplylaxis Investigators Prevention of venous thromboembolism in the acute treatment phase after spinal cord injury: a randomized, multicenter trial comparing low-dose heparin plus intermittent pneumatic compression with enoxaparin. J Trauma 2003; 54: 1116–1124.

R. *Chavko*   M.R. *Pinsky*

Functional haemodynamic monitoring

Cardiovascular insufficiency manifesting as circulatory shock is one of the most commonly encountered situations in the intensive care unit (ICU). Adequate delivery of oxygenated blood to tissues is only possible when there is sufficient amount not only of blood flow but also regulation of flow. Cardiac output is influenced by factors that alter preload, that alter myocardial contractility and those that alter afterload. Together with arterial tone, cardiac output is the primary determinant of arterial pressure defining organ blood flow. Physicians often begin their treatment of cardiovascular insufficiency states by assuming that the inappropriately low cardiac output can be raised by increasing preload. This gives rise to the time-honoured act of immediate volume resuscitation for all patients that present with circulatory shock. However, volume expansion will only increase cardiac output in that subset of patients who are preload responsive. Subjects with acute cor pulmonale from a massive pulmonary embolism or severe left ventricular failure of any cause will not only fail to increase cardiac output in response to volume expansion, but may demonstrate further cardiovascular decompensation. Furthermore, if arterial tone is markedly reduced, then arterial pressure may not increase with volume expansion despite an increase in cardiac output, thus minimizing the ability of the patient to increase organ blood flow, as the primary determinant of organ blood flow in circulatory shock states is organ perfusion pressure. Preload responsiveness is defined as increase in cardiac output as a reaction to infusing intravascular volume. Since the accuracy of measuring changes in cardiac output under clinical conditions is questionable, a threshold value of usually more than 15% increase in cardiac output is taken as a clinically relevant increase. In preload, non-responders cardiac output will not only fail to increase but may actually decrease in the setting of acute cor pulmonale and oxygen delivery to the tissues may decrease in both acute cor pulmonale and patients with pulmonary oedema. Thus, it is preferable to identify patients who are preload responsive and those who are not. If one can also define arterial tone, one can then develop a treatment philosophy that includes the appropriate use of volume expansion, vasopressor and inotropic agents. Two of the primary goals of haemodynamic monitoring are to identify the presence of circulatory shock and to guide specific goal-directed treatments. Recent advances in monitoring techniques and clinical trials support the rationale of applying 'functional' measures of cardiovascular performance that define specific treatment approaches, rather than just the measurement of static haemodynamic values that may reflect a variety of disease processes and their potential responsiveness to treatments. To a large extent, the failure of the pulmonary artery catheter to show any improved outcome from critical illness reflects this lack of goal-directed monitoring, in favour of focusing on the quality of the individual measured haemodynamic variables.

Traditional 'Static' Measures of Cardiovascular Status

Within certain limits the heart responds to increasing preload by augmentation in left ventricular stroke volume (SV). The relationship between left ventricular end-diastolic volume (EDV) and SV is known as the Frank–Starling relationship (Fig. 7.1). Inherent in its use in clinical medicine is the assumption that, in a fluid-responsive state, increases in left ventricular EDV will be associated with proportional increases in SV. The Frank–Starling formulation has been utilized in bedside haemodynamic monitoring in attempts to predict fluid responsiveness. The assumption being made is that if left ventricular EDV is reduced then the subject will be preload responsive and if left ventricular EDV is increased then they will not be preload responsive. Left ventricular EDV is difficult to measure at the bedside and nearly impossible to measure continually over time. However, surrogate measures that are presumed to reflect left ventricular EDV are usually used in applying Frank–Starling concepts to the management of the critically ill patient.

Most studies using this Frank–Starling construct have focused on surrogate measures of left ventricular EDV. Thus, investigators and clinicians alike have relied on estimates of left ventricular filling pressure to estimate left ventricular EDV and its response to therapeutic manoeuvres. In this

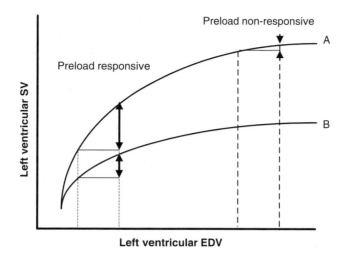

Figure 7.1 Frank–Starling relationship for normal heart (A) and a heart with decreased contractility (B). Equal increases In preload cause variable increases in SV relative to starting preload and contractility.

regard, balloon flotation pulmonary arterial catheterization allows for the measurement of pulmonary venous pressure near the inflow point of the left atrium by measuring the stop-flow pulmonary artery pressure by balloon occlusion, referred to as pulmonary artery occlusion pressure (P_{pao}). As a further reduction of this estimate, measures of right ventricular filling pressure can also be estimated by central venous pressure (CVP) or right atrial pressure (P_{ra}). There are a number of limitations to P_{pao} reflecting left ventricular EDV. First of all, P_{pao} is not the 'filling' pressure for the left ventricule. Even if P_{pao} represents left atrial pressure, P_{pao} correlates poorly with the presystolic rise in left ventricular end-diastolic pressure (EDP) caused by atrial systole. Atrial systole is responsible for a considerable part of left ventricular preload in subjects in normal sinus rhythm. Furthermore, P_{pao} does not take into account the amount of pericardial pressure on the outside of the heart that opposes left ventricular distension. Pericardial pressure is a major determinant of left ventricular distending pressure, and if pericardial pressure is markedly increased, as may occur with acute left or right ventricular over-distention, pulmonary hyperinflation and pericardial tamponade, estimates of left ventricular distending pressure made from P_{pao} measures alone will grossly underestimate true distending pressure. Finally, the relationship between P_{pao} and left ventricular EDV is neither linear nor constant over time. Under normal conditions, the relationship between left ventricular distending pressure and left ventricular EDV, referred to as left ventricular diastolic compliance, is curvilinear, with the left ventricular compliance markedly decreasing at larger EDV values. Left ventricular diastolic compliance also varies between and within subjects over time. Ischaemia immediately reduces left ventricular diastolic compliance, whereas nitrates increase it. Thus, neither the absolute P_{pao} value nor its change will reproducibly predict the absolute value or change in left ventricular EDP. Lastly, even if one knew accurately the baseline left ventricular EDV and its filling pressure, these data would not define left ventricular diastolic compliance, which itself may vary widely over time and for the same left ventricular EDV. Similarly, P_{ra} as an indicator of right ventricular preload is subject to similar limitations with an added deviation due to the possibility of unequal load on the ventricles.

Echocardiography more reliably estimates the left ventricular EDV as end-diastolic area (EDA). But since it does not measure left ventricular filling pressures, it does not allow one to assess left ventricular diastolic compliance. Static measures of left ventricular EDA reflect more closely the left ventricular EDV and their changes than do either P_{pao} or P_{ra}. Given this observation, it is surprising that neither P_{pao}, P_{ra} nor left ventricular EDA measures reliably predict preload responsiveness in haemodynamically unstable patients.[1-7] The reasons for this lack of correlation and the subsequent development of more functional measures of preload responsiveness are instructive in understanding not only cardiovascular physiology, but also the recent failures to define the utility of the pulmonary artery catheter when used in a protocolized fashion.

In a simplified model, preload would be represented by the 'filling pressure' P_{pao}, while SV would be represented by myofibril length, or left ventricular EDA. If the slope of the Frank–Starling curve were constant between and within subjects, one could predict the response to volume expansion using either P_{pao} or left ventricular EDA. However, changes in left ventricular compliance, impaired myocardial contraction or increased pericardial pressure, which can potentially change over a few heartbeats, provide for an infinite numbers of Frank–Starling curves and limit the usefulness of static measurements of filling pressure and SV in the ICU. Without knowing either the slope of the Frank–Starling curve or the effective left ventricular diastolic compliance, it is difficult, if not impossible, to predict the response to volume expansion even when one localizes the exact point on the Frank–Starling curve at which the heart is operating.[8]

Physiological Rationale for 'Functional' Haemodynamic Monitoring

Spontaneous respiration

The spontaneous ventilation-induced variation in blood pressure has been described since antiquity and is called *pulsus paradoxus*. 'Paradoxus' because the heartbeat was felt during deep inspiration but the peripheral pulse was not. In antiquity this was usually due to tuberculous pericarditis. To understand the effect of respiration on haemodynamic variables we need to be aware of the basics of cardiopulmonary physiology. Under normal conditions both the right and left ventricles operate on the steep portion of the Frank–Starling curve, such that relatively small changes in preload cause bigger changes in SV unless ventricular failure or hypervolaemia co-exist. The heart and intrathoracic great vessels can be imagined as a connected system of chambers with relatively compliant walls in which blood flows along pressure gradients. Contained in the relatively rigid thoracic cavity, the system is subjected to respiratory fluctuations of intrathoracic pressure relative to the compliance of surrounding structures and walls. The gradient propelling venous blood into the right heart stays constant during apnoea. However, during spontaneous inspiration, the diaphragm moves downwards and exerts two effects, both of which increase the gradient filling the right atrium. First, intrathoracic pressure decreases this is partly transmited into the chambers contained within the thorax, including the right atrium. At the same time, diaphragm descent increases intra-abdominal pressure by increasing the pressure in the abdominal inferior vena cava. Small increases in pressure gradient for venous return accelerate blood flow into the right heart and fill the right ventricle to a greater EDV. If the right ventricle is operating on the steep portion of the Frank–Starling curve, the effect is to markedly increase right ventricular SV. The left side of the heart sees the resulting transient surge in the pulmonary blood flow after a delay of 2–3 beats, which is the time needed for this extra blood to traverse the pulmonary circulation. In addition, during inspiration when right ventricular EDV increases, left ventricular diastolic compliance is reduced by the process of ventricular interdependence, making the phasic changes in left ventricular SV even greater than the flow variations would create on their own. Right ventricular over-distension limited by the limiting pericardium that augments the ventilation-associated interdependence is seen. The effect of spontaneous inspiration on systemic arterial pressure can thus be explained by the transient drop in left heart output owing to a decrease in left ventricular filling.

Changes opposite to those during inspiration take place during spontaneous expiration. As the diaphragm rises to its neutral position, intrathoracic pressure returns to its resting sub-atmospheric value. Right heart filling gradients are decreased and right ventricular EDV and right ventricular SV decrease to pre-inspiratory values. The intraventricular septum that had previously bulged into the left ventricle returns to its neutral position as left ventricular diastolic compliance returns to pre-inspiration values.

If the right and left ventricular SV variation is exaggerated, the respiratory variation in the arterial pressure may become pronounced and is termed *pulsus paradoxus*. Such conditions may arise if a deeper than normal inspiratory drop in intrathoracic pressure creates larger a gradient right ventricular filling (as in asthma exacerbation) or increased pericardial pressure allows for a stronger effect of ventricular interdependence (as in pericardial tamponade). If P_{ra} decreases during spontaneous inspiration, then this is *prima facie* evidence that the right ventricle can handle an increased volume load without going into failure, and presumably the subject is volume responsive. Unfortunately, the changes in arterial pressure reflect more ventricular interdependence than preload responsiveness, so they cannot be used to identify preload responsiveness.

In summary, both right- and left-sided end-diastolic and SVs change cyclically during normal respiration. Right ventricular SV and right heart output rise transiently during inspiration and drop during expiration but since both right and left heart pumps work in series, right-sided variations are followed by left ventricular SV and left heart output, respectively, with a phase shift.[9]

Positive-pressure ventilation

The observation that arterial blood pressure varies in phase with respiration during intermittent positive-pressure breathing is not new. An inspiratory increase in arterial pressure in heart failure patients has been termed 'reverse *pulsus paradoxus*' to stress the dissimilarity to the decline in blood pressure observed during spontaneous inspiration.[10] Since the left ventricle and aorta are intrathoracic structures, they are subjected to varying intrathoracic pressure during mechanical breath, with intrathoracic pressure increasing with inspiration. If left ventricular SV were not to change, however, then both arterial systolic and diastolic pressure would increase equally. This is the so-called 'square wave' response to a Valsalva manoeuvre in subjects with severe heart failure. However, it is possible for arterial pulse pressure (PP) to increase in such patients during inspiration, if the increase in intrathoracic pressure effectively unloads left ventricular ejection. Analysis of simultaneous PP waves from pulmonary artery and radial artery as a correlate of SV has shown that right and left ventricular SV change in opposite directions during positive-pressure ventilation. Inspiratory increases in left ventricular SV are accompanied by decreases in right ventricular SV with the reversal of these changes during expiration. Ventricular filling pressures change in the same direction as do SV changes. Echocardiographical studies confirmed that the changes in SV reflect proportional changes in right and left ventricular preload.[11] Presumably, the rise in intrathoracic pressure during positive-pressure inspiration reduces right ventricular preload. Since the transmission of airway pressure to the pleural space is only partial, dependent on both chest wall and lung compliance, the overall effects of positive-pressure breathing will be different among subjects with different lung and chest wall status.

Increasing intrathoracic pressure directly increases P_{ra}, as the right atrium is a highly compliant structure and transmits external pressures to its internal fluid. Increasing intrathoracic pressure increases P_{ra}, decreasing the pressure gradient for systemic venous return, decreasing right ventricular EDV and consequently right ventricular SV.[12,13] This is the exact opposite process to that seen during spontaneous inspiration.[14] Inflation of the lung displaces the diaphragm into the abdomen increasing intra-abdominal pressure. Since a significant portion of venous return flowing through the abdomen is pressurized, the effect of positive-pressure ventilation on venous return is often minimized.[15] Therefore, as in spontaneous inspiration, the diaphragm mitigates the expected decrease in right heart filling by simultaneously pressurizing the inferior vena cava. Right heart preload is not the only determinant of right ventricular SV affected by mechanical lung inflation. Although some pulmonary vessels are distended by the pull of surrounding structures with lung expansion, the net effect of inspiration is an increase in pulmonary vascular resistance (PVR) as small vessels in contact with alveolar air are squeezed by higher surrounding pressure and a resulting rise in right ventricular afterload causes a decrease in right ventricular SV.[16] The exception to this finding occurs when mechanical breaths re-expand collapsed alveoli reversing pre-existing hypoxic pulmonary vasoconstriction. However, the role of higher afterload in limiting the inspiratory right ventricular SV usually is overshadowed by the associated decrease in right ventricular preload.[17,18] In this manner, right ventricular SV periodically decreases with mechanical inspiration and the decrease in right heart output results, after two to three beats, in a decrease in left ventricular filling.[19]

Mechanical ventilation also directly alters left ventricular preload. An inspiration mechanically squeezes blood out of pulmonary veins into the left heart.[20] In contrast to the pulmonary vasculature, the aorta is not subjected to as much pressure transmission and with the increased intrathoracic pressure, pressure gradient-induced by the mechanical breath, the pressure gradient between left ventricle and aorta falls, effectively decreasing left ventricular afterload. Augmented inflow of blood into the left heart combines with lower left ventricular afterload to cause a transient increase in left ventricular SV.[21,22] However, the effect of afterload change is again minor[23,24] and the main reason why left ventricular SV is increased with mechanical inspiration is the increased amount of blood, ejected by the right ventricle during expiration, arriving in the left heart and the increased pulmonary venous flow. The decreases in left ventricular diastolic compliance caused by right ventricular dilatation through intraventricular interdependence are less pronounced during positive-pressure ventilation than with spontaneous respiration as right ventricular volumes usually decrease with mechanical respiration. Nevertheless, the right ventricular size can increase with mechanical inspiration if venous return is not impaired, as may occur with volume overload or increased intra-abdominal pressure, associated with increased PVR.

Mechanical expiration sees the turnaround of haemodynamic changes. Decrease in intrathoracic pressure allows the right ventricular preload to rise back to baseline thus reversing the inspiratory fall in right ventricular SV. Higher right heart output, however, will get to the left heart with a delay of pulmonary transition time and the left heart is being filled by lower pulmonary flow ejected from the right ventricle during mechanical inspiration at this time. Increase in left ventricular afterload from lowered intrathoracic pressure is another factor causing expiratory return of left ventricular SV to lower volume.

The effect of change in preload on either right or left ventricular SV is most pronounced when the heart operates at the steep portion of the Frank–Starling curve. If right ventricular SV variability and inflow of blood into the left heart is the most important determinant of left ventricular SV variability, there will be only minimal left ventricular SV change if right ventricular is not preload dependent. Conversely, even the presence of right ventricular SV variability does not warrant left ventricular SV variability since left ventricular may not be preload dependent.[25,26] Thus, magnitude of respiratory left ventricular SV changes is an indicator of biventricular preload dependence.[27] Accordingly, left ventricular SV variations are a true marker of overall cardiac preload responsiveness because the entire cardiac system (left and right) needs to be preload responsive for left ventricular SV variations to occur during positive-pressure ventilation.

Arterial blood pressure is a product of cardiac output and arterial tone. Selective changes in either will manifest themselves as a blood pressure change. Alterations in arterial tone generally take place over a longer time than one respiratory cycle and beat-to-beat variation in blood pressure can better be explained by varying left ventricular SV. Thus, the variations in blood pressure with respiration are caused by variations in cardiac output and left ventricular SV if we assume that heart rate (HR) stays relatively constant.

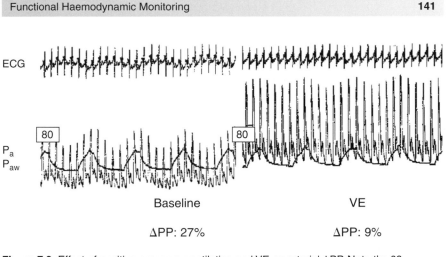

ECG

P_a
P_{aw}

Baseline   VE

ΔPP: 27%   ΔPP: 9%

Figure 7.2 Effect of positive-pressure ventilation and VE on arterial ΔPP. Note the 80 reference line reflects 80 mmHg for the P_a tracing, not the P_{aw} tracing, which is superimposed on the P_a tracing for illustrative purposes only. The amount of ΔPP is significantly reduced after VE (François Jardin: personal communication). ECG: electrocardiogram; P_a: arterial pressure; P_{aw}: airway pressure.

In summary SVs of both ventricles undergo cyclical changes during mechanical ventilation. Inspiration decreases preload to the right heart and results in decreased right heart output while left heart preload is boosted and causes a transient increase in left ventricular output and arterial pressure.[28] Mechanical expiration on the other hand allows for higher filling of the right ventricle and higher right heart output while lower flow into the left heart results in temporary decrease in left heart output and resulting drop in arterial pressure (Fig. 7.2).

Usefulness of 'Dynamic' Monitoring

All currently investigated methods of functional haemodynamic monitoring utilize modifications of the same concept. If the right heart is preload sensitive, then small variations in preload will trigger sizeable variations in right-sided output. Since preload is the most important determinant of left-sided output, right heart output variability will manifest as comparable variability in left heart preload and, therefore, left heart output provided the left ventricle is preload sensitive as well. The same change in preload does not always cause the same change in output depending on what part of the Frank–Starling curve that ventricle is operating on. As the ventricular diastolic dimensions stretch, the heart becomes less preload responsive. In other words, for the same reduction in right ventricular preload (due to pressure increase inside the chest) changes in right ventricular output will be greatest when the right ventricle is under filled and may show no effects if the right ventricle is overly distended. These cyclic haemodynamic responses can be measured and quantified as variations in cardiac chamber dimensions, volumes and their dependent variables. Variations in left ventricular output stemming from unequal SVs and resulting variations in arterial pressure and flows are among the most commonly investigated parameters.

Variations in Right Atrial Pressure

The erroneous assumption that CVP represents right ventricular EDV is frequently made. Let us assume that CVP actually does reflect right ventricular EDP. If the right ventricle is filling at low volumes, then a decrease in pericardial pressure, as occurs with spontaneous inspiration, will dilate this chamber and cause a decrease of pressure inside. If, on the other hand, the right ventricle fills at or beyond its stressed volume, then the distended right ventricular walls will not allow significant further dilatation of the chamber and pressure will not dip with spontaneous inspiration. Indeed, attempts have been made to differentiate between responders and non-responders by response of P_{ra} to intrathoracic pressure fluctuations with spontaneous breathing.[29,30] If sufficient spontaneous respiratory effort (as evidenced by a decrease in P_{pao} of more than 2 mmHg) lowers P_{ra} by more than 1 mmHg, subjects are expected to be fluid responsive. Magder and colleagues used this logic to predict preload responsiveness in spontaneously breathing subjects. A rise in cardiac output of more than 250 ml/min was observed with volume loading in 13 out of 14 such subjects who displayed such inspiration-associated decreases in P_{ra}. If good inspiratory effort does not produce such a measurable drop in P_{ra} then those subjects' cardiac output is probably not preload responsive.[29] Unfortunately, few patients in intensive care are breathing by a purely spontaneous effort, thus making this method less usable.[30]

Variations in Left Ventricular Stroke Volume

Due to the shape of the Frank–Starling curve, alterations in SV corresponding to the same absolute preload reduction will be highest in low preload states and smallest with high preload. Beaussier and colleagues indirectly verified variations in left heart output in humans on mechanical ventilation. Variation in velocity time integral, the indirect measure of left ventricular SV, corresponded to variation in aortic systolic blood pressure. After volume loading systolic pressure variation decreased and so did the variation in velocity time integral.[31] New technology capable of beat-to-beat measurements of left ventricular SV by analysis of invasive systolic arterial pressure wave using sophisticated algorithms (pulse contour analysis) can display SV variation (in per cent) as a ratio of difference between maximal and minimal to average systolic blood pressure in a floating window of the previous 30 s. The decrease in SV variation monitored online after volume challenge correlates well with accompanying decrease in systolic pressure variation measured offline.[32] This method has been correlated with fluid responsiveness, but with mixed results. In patients undergoing brain surgery SV variation of ≥9.5% reasonably identified subjects who would respond to subsequent small volume load by increase in left ventricular SV of at least 5%.[33] Similar association of increase in cardiac index (CI) after volume loading with SV variation decrease and baseline absolute SV variation percentage was observed in mechanically ventilated patients following cardiac surgery.[34] Unfortunately, the expected correlation of changes in SV or cardiac output after volume expansion with pulse contour derived changes in SV variation was not reproduced in another study of patients undergoing cardiac surgery.[35]

Variations in Systemic Arterial Blood Pressure (Systolic Pressure and Pulse Pressure)

The initial observations of systolic blood pressure variation during breathing noted that, in subjects with constrictive pericarditis, the peripheral pulse disappeared during inspiration, while the central heartbeat could still be felt. This phenomenon was referred to as 'pulsus paradoxus.' Arterial pulsus is quantified in mmHg, as the difference between maximal and minimal systolic blood pressure variation over a ventilatory cycle, whereas systolic blood pressure variation is quantified as the per cent change in systolic pressure during one mechanical breath divided by the mean systolic pressure. This systolic blood pressure variation can be divided into two separate components. If systolic pressure increases relative to apnoeic values, it is referred to as Δup. Decreases in systolic pressure relative to apnoeic values are referred to as Δdown. In hypovolaemic patients, Δdown is the main component of difference in systolic blood pressure and correlates with preload responsiveness since the magnitude of Δdown decreases after fluid resuscitation.[36] Inducing hypotension in mechanically ventilated dogs via bleeding or vasodilator infusion increased Δdown. Pizov and colleagues observed that while systolic blood pressure variation and particularly Δdown increased in both positive-pressure ventilation and haemorrhage the Δdown was considerably higher in haemorrhaged subjects. They concluded that the measurements of respiratory variation could be used to discern hypotension caused predominantly by hypovolaemia from hypotension of other aetiologies.[37] Both systolic blood pressure variation and Δdown increased in mechanically ventilated dogs bled gradually by up to 30% of blood volume.

Not surprisingly, systolic blood pressure variation and per cent systolic blood pressure variation correlated better to degree of haemorrhage than static haemodynamic indicators, such as CVP and mean arterial pressure (MAP). Following restoration of intravascular volume status all haemodynamic variables returned to their baseline[38] by decreasing the Δdown component of systolic blood pressure variation.[24] While Δdown is the main determinant of systolic blood pressure variation in hypovolaemia, the relative importance of Δup surfaces in ventricular failure and hypervolaemia. In both these states a ventricle is operating close to the 'flat portion' of its performance curve when minimal preload responsiveness also exists. Under these circumstances increase in SV are possible mainly by improvement in contractility or decrease in afterload. The ratio of Δup/Δdown increased dramatically and systolic blood pressure variation was mostly made of Δup with experimental acute ventricular failure and hypervolaemia.[23] Confirming the data in mechanically ventilated humans, the magnitude of systolic blood pressure variation and Δdown predicted changes in CI in response to volume expansion. These functional parameters (systolic blood pressurevariation and Δdown) successfully correlated to transesophageal echocardiographical indicators of preload in vascular surgery patients. Systolic blood pressure variation threshold of 12 mmHg identified subjects with findings of inadequate intravascular volume.[39] Another human study confirmed the ability of systolic blood pressure variation and Δdown to predict volume responsiveness in mechanically ventilated subjects that were made hypovolaemic by controlled haemorrhage and had volume subsequently replaced by intravenous (i.v.) fluids. Systolic blood pressure variation of 5 mmHg or less or Δdown of 2 mmHg or less appeared to be markers of adequate fluid resuscitation.[40] If variations in systolic blood pressure are high in subjects that are hypovolaemic and low in adequately expanded subjects, then the amount of baseline systolic blood pressure variation may predict the degree to which cardiac indices will drop with volume depletion or rise with repletion. Baseline systolic blood pressure variation was able to estimate how much cardiac output will drop as a result of controlled haemorrhage in mechanically ventilated human subjects. Pre-haemorrhage systolic blood pressure variation of ≤15 mmHg was identified as a predictor of a 20% or less drop in cardiac output after 500 ml bleeding. Systolic blood pressure variation of >15 mmHg on the other hand, as a marker of latent hypovolaemia, singled out the subjects in whom cardiac output would fall more than 20% with acute preload decrease.[41] Expanding the usefulness of functional indicators to predict response to volume expansion in low preload states, systolic blood pressure variation and Δdown proved to be good predictors in states where a combination of low afterload and preload is responsible for blood pressure decrease, such as in sepsis. Cutoff values of 10 mmHg in systolic blood pressure variation and 5 mmHg in Δdown were good predictors of increase in SV index (SVI) of 15% or more in response to volume expansion.[7]

Systolic blood pressure variation may not be the ideal indicator of SV variation. Even with no SV variation, systolic blood pressure variation could still be present as a direct transmission of changing intrathoracic pressure into a column of arterial blood. In support of this hypothesis, Denault et al.[42] showed that systolic blood pressure variation co-varied more with airway pressure than with changes in left ventricular EDA in intra-operative cardiac surgical patients. PP, the difference between systolic and diastolic arterial pressure, should escape this pressure superposition as both systolic and diastolic components are subjected to the same intrathoracic pressure fluctuation. Utilizing this concept it was shown that respiratory variation in PP (PPV or ΔPP) = PP_{max} at inspiration − PP_{min} at inspiration, and predicts the effect of volume loading on increase in CI of ≥15% better than systolic blood pressure variation in subjects with septic shock[2] (Fig. 7.3). ΔPP of more than 13% identified responders whereas lower ΔPP meant that CI increase would be lower than 15%. Interestingly, the authors noted that the magnitude of increase in CI in response to 500 ml fluid load was about the same as the magnitude of ΔPP at baseline. Considering that each mechanical inspiration causes increase in intrathoracic pressure comparable to that of

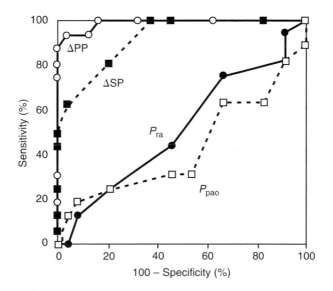

Figure 7.3 Receiver-operator characteristic for preload indicators predicting more than 15% increase in cardiac output after volume expansion with 500 ml of colloid in mechanically ventilated patients. ΔPP is a better predictor of volume responsiveness than ΔSP, but both dynamic indicators (ΔPP and ΔSP) are superior to static indicators (P_{ra} and P_{pao}). ΔSP: systolic pressure variability. Reprinted with permission from Michard *et al*. Am J Respir Crit Care 2000; 162: 134–138.

positive end-expiratory pressure (PEEP), but short lived, it should not be surprising that ΔPP at zero PEEP predicted the amount of drop in CI after adding $10\,cmH_2O$ PEEP in subjects with acute lung injury. If the PEEP-induced decrease in CI was $\geq 10\%$ then volume loading increased CI, and the increase correlated to both ΔPP on PEEP and fluid-induced change in ΔPP.[43] A similar correlation was documented for septic patients given fluid resuscitation.[2]

Variations in Velocities and Flows

Invasive blood pressure monitoring via arterial catheterization is required for dynamic PP monitoring methods and, although less invasive than pulmonary catheterization, it still remains an invasive procedure with risks of significant morbidity. A method that could evaluate respiratory changes in SVs without the potential for complications would be an attractive alternative. Measuring variations in blood flow assuming constant cross-sectional area could detect the same respiratory changes in left heart output as measuring variations in SV blood pressure does. Similarly to magnitude in baseline systolic blood pressure variation, baseline variation in peak aortic flow velocity, at the level of the aortic valve, of more than 12% identified mechanically ventilated humans in whom CI would rise by 15% or more in response to volume infusion.[44] Another method, infrared photo-plethysmography, allows continuous measurement of finger blood pressure, which has been shown to correspond to changes in blood pressure.[45] Applying this concept, a correlation between invasively measured ΔPP and non-invasive ΔPP was found.[46]

Summary

Identification of fluid responsiveness in the ICU can avoid risky manoeuvres or volume infusion in subjects who may not benefit from higher preload. Traditional 'static' measurements of right atrial pressure (RAP), pulmonary artery occlusive pressure (PAOP) and right ventricular EDV are still widely used to assess fluid responsiveness despite having produced conflicting data in studies.

Mechanical ventilation induces cyclic intrathoracic pressure changes and often constant intrathoracic pressure increase when PEEP is used. Variable intrathoracic pressure influences filling pressures of both ventricles' preload, the major determinant of SV. Wavering right heart preload transfers into variable right ventricular SV if right ventricular is preload responsive. Variable right ventricular SV changes left ventricular SV, with a delay of pulmonary transition time, in the same direction if the left heart is preload responsive as well. The presence of left ventricular SV variability thus signifies preload dependence of both ventricles. Cardiac outputs of both ventricles move in the same direction as SVs since HR variability is much smaller. Variable outputs can be measured indirectly as differences in peak aortic blood flow velocity, systolic blood pressure, PP or integrals of PP wave. The magnitude of variability corresponds to the degree of preload dependence. The variability of haemodynamic indicators uniformly increases with hypovolaemia and decreases with volume expansion. Furthermore, the amount of baseline variability can be used to estimate the rise of SV, cardiac output and their indices in response to volume expansion, to permit titration of volume expansion (VE) and to identify low cardiac output associated with low preload. Respiratory changes in haemodynamics ('dynamic' indicators) therefore provide better clues to fluid resuscitation-induced haemodynamics (Fig. 7.4).

Use of dynamic indicators in assessing hypovolaemia is currently limited to sedated and mechanically ventilated patients at best as most studies examined sedated subjects on positive-pressure ventilation. Inconsistency of effort in spontaneous breathing (and amount of resulting preload change) is one of the major factors deterring quantification of its effect. Similarly,

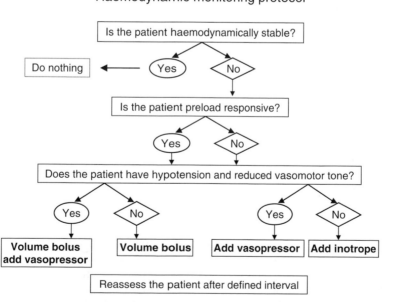

Figure 7.4 Logistic algorithm for treating haemodynamic instability. Based on the answers to three sequential questions, one may give nothing, volume, volume plus pressor, pressor or inotropic agents. Clearly, volume expansion is the first line of treatment in patients that are preload responsive. However, vasopressor agents are added in patients with reduced vasomotor tone. In contrast, inotropic and/or vasopressor agents are used initially in haemodynamically unstable patients who are not preload responsive.

mechanical tidal volume and breathing rate must be held constant as variability will arguably cause unequal intrathoracic pressure swings and possibly increase intrinsic PEEP.[47] Presence of baseline unpredictably variable SV changes, such as in atrial arrhythmias, is another situation in which assessing the effect of intrathoracic pressure-induced preload changes is impossible.

Finally and most importantly, it has not been demonstrated that therapy guided by dynamic indicators provides survival advantage. In other words, diagnosis of biventricular preload dependence in the presence of circulatory insufficiency does not necessarily mean that increasing preload will alter prognosis.

References

1. Reuse C, Vincent JL, Pinsky MR. Measurements of right ventricular volumes during fluid challenge. Chest 1990; 98: 1450–1454.
2. Michard F, Boussat S, Chemla D, Anguel N, Mercat A, Lecarpentier Y, Richard C, Pinsky MR, Teboul JL. Relation between respiratory changes in arterial pulse pressure and fluid responsiveness in septic patients with acute circulatory failure. Am J Respir Crit Care Med 2000; 162: 134–138.
3. Calvin JE, Driedger AA, Sibbald WJ. The haemodynamic effect of rapid fluid infusion in critically ill patients. Surgery 1981; 90: 61–76.
4. Tousignant CP, Walsh F, Mazer CD. The use of transesophageal echocardiography for preload assessment in critically ill patients. Anesth Analg 2000; 90: 351–355.
5. Diebel LN, Wilson RF, Tagett MG, Kline RA. End-diastolic volume. A better indicator of preload in the critically ill. Arch Surg 1992; 127: 817–821.
6. Diebel L, Wilson RF, Heins J, Larky H, Warsow K, Wilson S. End-diastolic volume versus pulmonary artery wedge pressure in evaluating cardiac preload in trauma patients. J Trauma 1994; 37: 950–955.
7. Tavernier B, Makhotine O, Lebuffe G, Dupont J, Scherpereel P. Systolic pressure variation as a guide to fluid therapy in patients with sepsis-induced hypotension. Anesthesiology 1998; 89: 1313–1321.
8. Michard F, Teboul JL. Using heart–lung interactions to assess fluid responsiveness during mechanical ventilation. Crit Care 2000; 4: 282–289.
9. Pinsky MR. Hemodynamic effects of ventilation and ventilatory maneuvers. In: Scharf SM, Pinsky MR, Magder S (eds) Respiratory–Circulatory Interactions in Health and Disease. New York: Marcel Dekker, 2001; 183–209.
10. Massumi RA, Mason DT, Vera Z, Zelis R, Otero J, Amsterdam EA. Reversed pulsus paradoxus. New Engl J Med 1973; 13(289): 1272–1275.
11. Jardin F, Farcot JC, Gueret P, Prost JF, Ozier Y, Bourdarias JP. Cyclic changes in arterial pulse during respiratory support. Circulation 1983; 68: 266–274.
12. Morgan BC, Martin WE, Hornbein TF, Crawford EW, Guntheroth WG. Hemodynamic effects of intermittent positive pressure ventilation. Anesthesiology 1966; 27: 584–590.
13. Scharf SM, Brown R, Saunders N, Green LH. Hemodynamic effects of positive-pressure inflation. J Appl Physiol 1980; 49: 124–131.
14. Wise RA, Robotham JL, Summer WR. Effects of spontaneous ventilation on the circulation. Lung 1981; 159: 175–186.

15. Takata M, Robotham JL. Effects of inspiratory diaphragmatic descent on inferior vena caval venous return. J Appl Physiol 1992; 72: 597–607.
16. Lopez-Muniz R, Stephens NL, Bromberger-Barnea B, Permutt S, Riley RL. Critical closure of pulmonary vessels analyzed in terms of Starling resistor model. J Appl Physiol 1968; 24: 625–635.
17. Permutt S, Wise RA, Brower RG. How changes in pleural and alveolar pressure cause changes in afterload and preload. In: Scharf SM, Cassidy SS (eds) Heart–Lung Interactions in Health and Disease. New York: Marcel Dekker, 1989; 243–250.
18. Theres H, Binkau J, Laule M, Heinze R, Hundertmark J, Blobner M, Erhardt W, Baumann G, Stangl K. Phase-related changes in right ventricular cardiac output under volume-controlled mechanical ventilation with positive end-expiratory pressure. Crit Care Med 1999; 27: 953–958.
19. Scharf SM, Brown R, Saunders N, Green LH. Hemodynamic effects of positive-pressure inflation. J Appl Physiol 1980; 49: 124–131.
20. Brower R, Wise RA, Hassapoyannes C, Bronberger-Barnea B, Permutt S. Effects of lung inflation on lung blood volume and pulmonary venous flow. J Appl Physiol 1985; 58: 954–963.
21. Pinsky MR, Matuschak GM, Klain M. Determinants of cardiac augmentation by elevations in intrathoracic pressure. J Appl Physiol 1985; 58: 1189–1198.
22. Fessler HE, Brower RG, Wise RA, Permutt S. Mechanism of reduced left ventricular afterload by systolic and diastolic positive pleural pressure. J Appl Physiol 1988; 65: 1244–1250.
23. Pizov R, Ya'ari Y, Perel A. The arterial pressure waveform during acute ventricular failure and synchronized external chest compression. Anesth Analg 1989; 68: 150–156.
24. Szold A, Pizov R, Segal E, Perel A. The effect of tidal volume and intravascular volume state on systolic pressure variation in ventilated dogs. Intens Care Med 1989; 15: 368–371.
25. Magder S. The cardiovascular management of the critically ill patients. In: Pinsky MR (ed.) Applied Cardiovascular Physiology. Berlin: Springer, 1997; 28–35.
26. Guyton AC. Textbook of Medical Physiology, 8th ed. Philadelphia: WB Saunders, 1991.
27. Michard F, Teboul JL. Respiratory changes in arterial pressure in mechanically ventilated patients. In: Vincent JL (ed.) Yearbook of Intensive Care and Emergency Medicine. Berlin: Springer, 2000; 696–704.
28. Luce JM. The cardiovascular effects of mechanical ventilation and positive end-expiratory pressure. J Am Med Assoc 1984; 10(252): 807–811.
29. Magder S, Georgiadis G, Tuck C. Respiratory variations in right atrial pressure predict the response to fluid challenge. J Crit Care 1992; 7: 76–85.
30. Magder S, Lagonidis D. Effectiveness of albumin versus normal saline as a test of volume responsiveness in post-cardiac surgery patients. J Crit Care 1999; 14: 164–171.
31. Beaussier M, Coriat P, Perel A, Lebret F, Kalfon P, Chemla D, Lienhart A, Viars P. Determinants of systolic pressure variation in patients ventilated after vascular surgery. J Cardiothor Vascul Anesth 1995; 9: 547–551.
32. Reuter DA, Felbinger TW, Kilger E, Schmidt C, Lamm P, Goetz AE. Optimizing fluid therapy in mechanically ventilated patients after cardiac surgery by on-line monitoring of left ventricular stroke volume variations. Comparison with aortic systolic pressure variations. Brit J Anaesth 2002; 88: 124–126.

33. Berkenstadt H, Margalit N, Hadani M, Friedman Z, Segal E, Villa Y, Perel A. Stroke volume variation as a predictor of fluid responsiveness in patients undergoing brain surgery. Anesth Analg 2001; 92: 984–989.

34. Reuter DA, Felbinger TW, Schmidt C, Kilger E, Goedje O, Lamm P, Goetz AE. Stroke volume variations for assessment of cardiac responsiveness to volume loading in mechanically ventilated patients after cardiac surgery. Intensive Care Med 2002; 28: 392–398.

35. Wiesenack C, Prasser C, Rodig G, Keyl C. Stroke volume variation as an indicator of fluid responsiveness using pulse contour analysis in mechanically ventilated patients. Anesth Analg 2003; 96: 1254–1257.

36. Coyle JP, Teplick RS, Michael CL, Davison JK. Respiratory variations in systemic arterial pressure as an indicator of volume status. Anesthesiology 1983; 59: A53.

37. Pizov R, Ya'ari Y, Perel A. Systolic pressure variation is greater during haemorrhage than during sodium nitroprusside-induced hypotension in ventilated dogs. Anesth Analg 1988; 67: 170–174.

38. Perel A, Pizov R, Cotev S. Systolic blood pressure variation is a sensitive indicator of hypovolaemia in ventilated dogs subjected to graded haemorrhage. Anesthesiology 1987; 67: 498–502.

39. Coriat P, Vrillon M, Perel A, Baron JF, Le Bret F, Saada M, Viars P. A comparison of systolic blood pressure variations and echocardiographic estimates of end-diastolic left ventricular size in patients after aortic surgery. Anesth Analg 1994; 78: 46–53.

40. Rooke GA, Schwid HA, Shapira Y. The effect of graded haemorrhage and intravascular volume replacement on systolic pressure variation in humans during mechanical and spontaneous ventilation. Anesth Analg 1995; 80: 925–932.

41. Ornstein E, Eidelman LA, Drenger B, Elami A, Pizov R. Systolic pressure variation predicts the response to acute blood loss. J Clin Anesth 1998; 10: 137–140.

42. Denault AY, Gasior TA, Gorcsan III J, Mandarino WA, Deneault LG, Pinsky MR. Determinants of aortic pressure variation during positive-pressure ventilation in man. Chest 1999; 116: 176–186.

43. Michard F, Chemla D, Richard C, Wysocki M, Pinsky MR, Lecarpentier Y, Teboul JL. Clinical use of respiratory changes in arterial pulse pressure to monitor the haemodynamic effects of PEEP. Am J Respir Crit Care Med 1999; 159: 935–939.

44. Feissel M, Michard F, Mangin I, Ruyer O, Faller JP, Teboul JL. Respiratory changes in aortic blood velocity as an indicator of fluid responsiveness in ventilated patients with septic shock. Chest 2001; 119: 867–873.

45. Imholz BP, Wieling W, van Montfrans GA, Wesseling KH. Fifteen years experience with finger arterial pressure monitoring: assessment of the technology. Cardiovasc Res 1998; 38: 605–616.

46. Michard F, Mercat A, Chemla D, Richard C, Teboul, JL. Non invasive assessment of respiratory changes in arterial pulse pressure by infrared photoplethysmography in mechanically ventilated patients. Am J Respir Crit Care Med 1999; 159: A520.

47. Parry-Jones AJD, Pittman JAL. Arterial pressure and stroke volume variability as measurements for cardiovascular optimization. Int J Intensive Care 2003; 10: 67–72.

J.-L. Vincent

CHAPTER

8

Sepsis and the use of Xigris®

Sepsis, the most common disease process encountered in the critically ill population, has been, and continues to be, the subject of vast amounts of research at all levels from minute changes at the cellular level through to clinical therapeutics. This is an important field, with considerable associated morbidity, mortality and costs. Attempts to understand the mechanisms underlying the disease and hence to find an effective treatment have been rewarded with the development of drotrecogin alfa (activated), a recombinant form of the natural protein activated protein C (APC), marketed under the name Xigris® (Eli Lilly, Indianapolis, USA). This drug has been shown to improve outcomes in patients with severe sepsis and septic shock and will be the focus of this review.

Sepsis Pathogenesis

The importance of coagulation

The pathogenesis of sepsis is complex, involving multiple cells and mediators, all interacting to produce a network of interacting host inflammatory pathways. One such interacting pathway involves the endothelium and the coagulation system.[1,2] Early in the septic process, coagulation is activated by tissue factor, exposed on the surface of endothelial cells after stimulation with endotoxin[3] or pro-inflammatory mediators including interleukin-1 (IL-1), tumour necrosis factor (TNF) and platelet-activating factor (PAF).[4] Coagulation may also be initiated via contact system activation as a result of endotoxin, although the precise role of this pathway is unclear.[5] By whatever pathway, the end result is the conversion of prothrombin to thrombin, a protein with multiple functions within the coagulation system. In addition to its important procoagulant properties, thrombin also helps control coagulation by binding thrombomodulin, which is expressed on the endothelial cell surface, via the same binding site that is used by fibrinogen, platelets, and factor V, so that these functions are blocked.[6] The thrombin–thrombomodulin complex activates protein C in a process that is enhanced when protein C is bound to the endothelial cell protein C receptor (EPCR).[7–9] APC has several anticoagulant functions including the degradation of factors Va and VIIIa, with inhibition of thrombin generation.[10] APC also promotes fibrinolysis by inhibiting plasminogen activator inhibitor-1 (PAI-1) and thrombin activatable fibrinolysis inhibitor (TAFI),[11,12] and reduces tissue factor expression.[13]

In sepsis, the normal inhibitory mechanisms of coagulation are depressed, with reduced levels of antithrombin and protein C,[14] and after a brief period of activation, the fibrinolytic system is suppressed by release of PAI-1. Ongoing coagulation activity reduces platelet levels and coagulation factors, and there is a resultant procoagulant state. This may lead to the formation of microvascular thrombi, disturbing the local microcirculation, and potentially promoting the development of organ dysfunction.

While the inflammatory response is involved in the development of the abnormal procoagulant state during sepsis, the reverse is also true and many coagulation proteins are themselves actively involved in the inflammatory process. For example, thrombin induces the expression of various endothelial adhesion factors including E-selectin, P-selectin, and PAF,[6,15,16] and increases cytokine synthesis, by its interactions with protease-activated receptors (PARs),[17,18] and protein C, which is down-regulated in sepsis, has anti-inflammatory properties, inhibiting TNF production and neutrophil adhesion via selectins (see below).[19]

As the complex interactions between the coaguation and inflammatory systems were unravelled, studies were begun to determine whether manipulation of any of the coagulation factors could be of therapeutic value in sepsis.

Anti-inflammatory properties of activated protein C

In addition to its effects in the coagulation system, APC has indirect anti-inflammatory effects related to its inhibition of thrombin, but also has direct anti-inflammatory effects, including reducing nuclear translocation of nuclear factor-κB (NF-κB) with a resultant fall in synthesis of cytokines,[20] and reducing leukocyte adhesion and activation.[19,21] The exact mechanisms underlying these effects are uncertain, but studies have shown that all APC-induced protective genes, including the immunomod-ulatory monocyte chemoattractant protein-1 (MCP-1), occurred as the result of PAR-1 signalling.[22] APC also has anti-apoptotic activity, prob-ably mediated by the interaction between APC–EPCR and PARs.[2,22,23]

APC

The rationale behind the clinical trials

Protein C levels are reduced in patients with sepsis, and persistently reduced levels are associated with increased morbidity and mortal-ity.[14,24,25] In addition, case reports and small open-label studies suggested that protein C replacement can reduce morbidity and mortality in patients with *purpura fulminans* due to meningococcal disease.[26–29] However, the reduced activity of APC seen in sepsis is not just related to the reduced levels of protein C; several other factors are involved including the down-regulation of thrombomodulin and EPCR in sepsis, reducing the ability to activate protein C.[30–34] If the protein C cannot be converted to APC, simply replenishing protein C levels may, therefore, not provide as great an effect as if APC is given directly.

Preclinical studies were thus conducted with APC. In a baboon model of bacteremia[35] and a rabbit model of endotoxic shock,[36] APC administra-tion improved survival. In addition, blockade of protein C activation with a monoclonal antibody increased mortality.[35] These encouraging preclini-cal studies paved the way for clinical trials.

Clinical studies

A recombinant form of APC (drotrecogin alfa [activated]) was developed, and an initial phase II clinical trial in 131 patients with severe sepsis[37] showed that the drug was well-tolerated, and treated patients showed a dose-dependent reduction in D-dimer and IL-6 levels and a trend towards reduced mortality. A phase III clinical trial followed with results that led to the licensing of this drug for the direct treatment of patients with severe sepsis. The multicentre, randomized, controlled (PROWESS) study,[38] con-ducted between July 1998 and June 2000, involved 1690 patients from 164 centres in 11 countries, and was stopped at the second interim analy-sis as the beneficial effects on outcome became clear. Patients treated with 24 µg/kg/h of drotrecogin alfa (activated) for 96 h had a 6.1% absolute reduction in the relative risk of death at 28 days (30.8% placebo versus 24.7% treatment, $P = 0.005$), giving a reduction in the relative risk of death of 19.4% (95% confidence interval, 6.6–30.5%) for treatment with drotrecogin alfa (activated); that is 16 patients need to be treated to save one additional life. Since the original study publication, further analysis has demonstrated the beneficial effects of this drug on organ function, with a reduction in cardiovascular dysfunction in treated patients compared to placebo ($P = 0.022$), a faster resolution of cardiovascular ($P = 0.009$) and respiratory ($P = 0.009$) dysfunction, and a slower onset of haematological ($P = 0.041$) dysfunction.[39] Importantly, too, long-term follow-up data of the 28-day survivors from the PROWESS study show that the beneficial effects of treatment are maintained over time.[40] There was a suggestion that less severely ill patients may benefit less from drotrecogin alfa (activated), and indeed, a recent study assessing its use in patients with a lower risk of death (ADministration of DRotrecogin alfa [activated] in Early Severe Sepsis, ADDRESS) has been recently discontinued after the interim analysis. Indeed, patients with lower APACHE II scores do not show the same improved survival (unpublished data). The drug is therefore licensed only for the treatment of patients with severe sepsis and septic shock at a high risk of death, defined differently by the various licensing authorities; for example, APACHE score greater than 24 (USA), two or more sepsis-associated organ dysfunctions (Europe). In such patients it should be given early, as there seems to be a greater survival advantage in patients receiving drotrecogin alfa (activated) early after the onset of sepsis-related organ failure.[41]

As expected by the nature of APC, bleeding events are more common in patients treated with drotrecogin alfa (activated), but these are largely related to invasive procedures. In a study evaluating all reported use of this drug so far (2786 adult patients with severe sepsis enrolled in all phase 2 and 3 clinical trials), serious bleeding events occurred during the infusion period in 2.8% of patients and during the 28-day study period in 5.3% of patients.[42] Of the bleeding events during the infusion period, 43% were procedure related. Fatal serious bleeding events during the infusion period occurred in 0.4% of cases, and intracranial haemorrhage events during the infusion period occurred in 0.6% of patients. Ten out of the 16 intracranial haemorrhage events occurring during the study drug infusion period were associated with severe thrombocytopaenia (platelet count $\leq 30,000 \times 10^6$/l) and/or meningitis. There do not appear to be any other safety concerns with the use of drotrecogin alfa (activated).

The PROWESS study included only adult patients, but drotrecogin alfa (activated) appears to have similar pharmacokinetics, pharmacodynamic effects and safety profile in children.[43] A randomized controlled trial is currently under way to assess its effects on outcomes in this group of patients.

Practical considerations

Drotrecogin alfa (activated) cannot be used to replace basic resuscitation in the patient with severe sepsis. Adequate fluids and vasopressor agents must be given as required, and an infectious focus must be sought and treated with appropriate antibiotics and surgery as necessary. Other strategies recently shown to improve outcome, including careful control of blood sugar levels[44] and moderate doses of corticosteroids in patients with septic shock,[45] should now also be included in the sepsis-treatment package.

In the ideal world, all patients with severe sepsis should be considered for treatment with drotrecogin alfa (activated). One key limitation to this practice is that of expense: APC is an expensive drug at around 7500 euros/patient, but in cost-effectiveness studies it compares favourably with other well-accepted intensive care interventions, especially when restricted to more severely ill patients[46–49] and has been recommended as part of standard of care in modern critical healthcare systems.[50] Due to its increased risk of bleeding events, drotrecogin alfa (activated) is con-traindicated in patients at high risk of bleeding and care should be taken in certain other groups of patients (Table 8.1). In addition, it is recom-mended that treatment should be stopped 2 h prior to any surgical or inva-sive procedure and recommenced 2 (for minor procedures, e.g. chest tube insertion, central venous catheterization, etc.) to 12 (for major surgery) hours after the procedure is completed.[51]

Table 8.1 Absolute and relative contraindications to treatment with drotrecogin alfa (activated)

Absolute contraindications	Relative contraindications

• Active internal bleeding
• Trauma with an increased risk of life-threatening bleeding (e.g. to liver, spleen, etc.)
• Central nervous system (CNS) factors
  – Presence of an epidural catheter
  – Recent haemorrhagic stroke (3 months)
  – Recent CNS surgery/head trauma (2 months)
  – Intracranial mass or evidence of cerebral herniation
	• Abnormal coagulation
	  – Bleeding diathesis
	  – Platelet count <30,000 × 10⁶/l
	  – Very prolonged International Normalized Ratio (INR) >3.0
	  – Full heparin therapy
	  – Recent thrombolytic or glycoprotein IIb/IIIa therapy
	• Significant risk of bleeding
	  – Polytrauma
	  – Intracranial arteriovenous malformation or aneurysm
	  – Active gastric ulcer
	  – Oesophageal varices
	• Recent (within 3 months) ischaemic stroke

The Future

The development and licensing of the first immunomodulating drug to be shown to directly influence outcome from sepsis has been a huge advance in sepsis therapeutics. However, many questions remain unanswered. For example, as other immunomodulatory drugs are shown to be effective, where will they fit into the picture? It is quite possible that patients will benefit most from a cocktail of drugs, as is often the case with multisystem conditions such as cancer. But how will the physician decide which patient should receive which drug, or should they receive several, and if so together or one after the other? Will the effects be additive or synergistic, so doses could/should be reduced if given together? Will side effect profiles increase if more than one drug is given simultaneously? And will patients/hospitals/society be able to afford these often expensive drugs? These are just some of the many issues that require further study in this exciting field. Already a disease staging system, the PIRO (Predisposition; Insult; Response; Organ disfunction),[52] similar to the tumour, nodes, metastases (TNM) system for cancer patients, has been suggested and is being developed for use to characterize patients with sepsis; this will help to guide therapeutic decisions and monitor patient response to treatment. As further progress is made in this field, some of these complex issues will be resolved, and doubtless others will emerge – this is an exciting and rapidly advancing field and the development of drotrecogin alfa (activated), Xigris®, has given new impetus and encouragement to all involved in the care of the patient with sepsis.

References

1. Vincent JL. Microvascular endothelial dysfunction: a renewed appreciation of sepsis pathophysiology. Crit Care 2001; 5: S1–S5.
2. Levi M, Van der Poll T. The central role of the endothelium in the crosstalk between coagulation and inflammation in sepsis. Adv Sepsis 2004; 3: 91–97.
3. Franco RF, de Jonge E, Dekkers PE et al. The in vivo kinetics of tissue factor messenger RNA expression during human endotoxemia: relationship with activation of coagulation. Blood 2000; 96: 554–559.
4. Todoroki H, Higure A, Okamoto K et al. Possible role of platelet-activating factor in the in vivo expression of tissue factor in neutrophils. J Surg Res 1998; 80: 149–155.
5. Levi M, Keller TT, van Gorp E, ten Cate H. Infection and inflammation and the coagulation system. Cardiovasc Res 2003; 60: 26–39.
6. Esmon CT. The normal role of activated protein C in maintaining homeostasis and its relevance to critical illness. Crit Care 2001; 5: S7–S12.
7. Taylor Jr FB, Peer GT, Lockhart MS, Ferrell G, Esmon CT. Endothelial cell protein C receptor plays an important role in protein C activation in vivo. Blood 2001; 97: 1685–1688.
8. Stearns-Kurosawa DJ, Kurosawa S, Mollica JS, Ferrell GL, Esmon CT. The endothelial cell protein C receptor augments protein C activation by the

thrombin–thrombomodulin complex. Proc Natl Acad Sci USA 1996; 93: 10212–10216.

9. Xu J, Esmon NL, Esmon CT. Reconstitution of the human endothelial cell protein C receptor with thrombomodulin in phosphatidylcholine vesicles enhances protein C activation. J Biol Chem 1999; 274: 6704–6710.

10. Esmon CT. The regulation of natural anticoagulant pathways. Science 1987; 235: 1348–1352.

11. Krishnamurti C, Young GD, Barr CF, Colleton CA, Alving BM. Enhancement of tissue plasminogen activator-induced fibrinolysis by activated protein C in endotoxin-treated rabbits. J Lab Clin Med 1991; 118: 523–530.

12. Bajzar L, Nesheim ME, Tracy PB. The profibrinolytic effect of activated protein C in clots formed from plasma is TAFI-dependent. Blood 1996; 88: 2093–2100.

13. Shua F, Kobayashia H, Fukudomeb K, Tsuneyoshib N, Kimotob M, Teraoa T. Activated protein C suppresses tissue factor expression on U937 cells in the endothelial protein C receptor-dependent manner. FEBS Lett 2000; 477: 208–212.

14. Fourrier F, Chopin C, Goudemand J et al. Septic shock, multiple organ failure, and disseminated intravascular coagulation. Compared patterns of antithrombin III, protein C, and protein S deficiencies. Chest 1992; 101: 816–823.

15. Vercellotti GM, Wickham NW, Gustafson KS, Yin HQ, Hebert M, Jacob HS. Thrombin-treated endothelium primes neutrophil functions: inhibition by platelet-activating factor receptor antagonists. J Leukoc Biol 1989; 45: 483–490.

16. Kaplanski G, Fabrigoule M, Boulay V et al. Thrombin induces endothelial type II activation *in vitro*: IL-1 and TNF-alpha-independent IL-8 secretion and E-selectin expression. J Immunol 1997; 158: 5435–5441.

17. Naldini A, Carney DH, Pucci A, Pasquali A, Carraro F. Thrombin regulates the expression of proangiogenic cytokines via proteolytic activation of protease-activated receptor-1. Gen Pharmacol 2000; 35: 255–259.

18. Szaba FM, Smiley ST. Roles for thrombin and fibrin(ogen) in cytokine/chemokine production and macrophage adhesion *in vivo*. Blood 2002; 99: 1053–1059.

19. Grinnell BW, Hermann RB, Yan SB. Human protein C inhibits selectin-mediated cell adhesion: role of unique fucosylated oligosaccharide. Glycobiology 1994; 4: 221–225.

20. White B, Schmidt M, Murphy C et al. Activated protein C inhibits lipopolysaccharide-induced nuclear translocation of nuclear factor kappaB (NF-kappaB) and tumour necrosis factor alpha (TNF-alpha) production in the THP-1 monocytic cell line. Br J Haematol 2000; 110: 130–134.

21. Murakami K, Okajima K, Uchiba M et al. Activated protein C attenuates endotoxin-induced pulmonary vascular injury by inhibiting activated leukocytes in rats. Blood 1996; 87: 642–647.

22. Riewald M, Petrovan RJ, Donner A, Mueller BM, Ruf W. Activation of endothelial cell protease activated receptor 1 by the protein C pathway. Science 2002; 296: 1880–1882.

23. Mosnier LO, Griffin JH. Inhibition of staurosporine-induced apoptosis of endothelial cells by activated protein C requires protease activated receptor-1 and endothelial cell protein C receptor. Biochem J 2003; 373: 65–70.

24. Lorente JA, Garcia-Frade LJ, Landin L et al. Time course of hemostatic abnormalities in sepsis and its relation to outcome. Chest 1993; 103: 1536–1542.

25. Fisher Jr CJ, Yan SB. Protein C levels as a prognostic indicator of outcome in sepsis and related diseases. Crit Care Med 2000; 28: S49–S56.

26. Rivard GE, David M, Farrell C, Schwarz HP. Treatment of purpura fulminans in meningococcemia with protein C concentrate. J Pediatr 1995; 126: 646–652.

27. Ettingshausen CE, Veldmann A, Beeg T, Schneider W, Jager G, Kreuz W. Replacement therapy with protein C concentrate in infants and adolescents with meningococcal sepsis and purpura fulminans. Semin Thromb Hemost 1999; 25: 537–541.

28. Rintala E, Kauppila M, Seppala OP *et al*. Protein C substitution in sepsis-associated purpura fulminans. Crit Care Med 2000; 28: 2373–2378.

29. White B, Livingstone W, Murphy C, Hodgson A, Rafferty M, Smith OP. An open-label study of the role of adjuvant hemostatic support with protein C replacement therapy in purpura fulminans-associated meningococcemia. Blood 2000; 96: 3719–3724.

30. Redl H, Schlag G, Schiesser A, Davies J. Thrombomodulin release in baboon sepsis: its dependence on the dose of Escherichia coli and the presence of tumor necrosis factor. J Infect Dis 1995; 171: 1522–1527.

31. Moore KL, Esmon CT, Esmon NL. Tumor necrosis factor leads to the internalization and degradation of thrombomodulin from the surface of bovine aortic endothelial cells in culture. Blood 1989; 73: 159–165.

32. Speiser W, Kapiotis S, Kopp CW *et al*. Effect of intradermal tumor necrosis factor-alpha-induced inflammation on coagulation factors in dermal vessel endothelium. An *in vivo* study of human skin biopsies. Thromb Haemost 2001; 85: 362–367.

33. MacGregor IR, Perrie AM, Donnelly SC, Haslett C. Modulation of human endothelial thrombomodulin by neutrophils and their release products. Am J Respir Crit Care Med 1997; 155: 47–52.

34. Faust SN, Levin M, Harrison OB *et al*. Dysfunction of endothelial protein C activation in severe meningococcal sepsis. New Engl J Med 2001; 345: 408–416.

35. Taylor FB, Chang A, Esmon CT, D'Angelo A, Vigano-D'Angelo S, Blick KE. Protein C prevents the coagulopathic and lethal effects of *E. coli* in the baboon. J Clin Invest 1987; 79: 918–924.

36. Roback MG, Stack AM, Thompson C, Brugnara C, Schwarz HP, Saladino RA. Activated protein C concentrate for the treatment of meningococcal endotoxin shock in rabbits. Shock 1998; 9: 138–142.

37. Bernard GR, Ely EW, Wright TJ *et al*. Safety and dose relationship of recombinant human activated protein C for coagulopathy in severe sepsis. Crit Care Med 2001; 29: 2051–2059.

38. Bernard GR, Vincent JL, Laterre PF *et al*. Efficacy and safety of recombinant human activated protein C for severe sepsis. New Engl J Med 2001; 344: 699–709.

39. Vincent JL, Angus DC, Artigas A *et al*. Effects of drotrecogin alfa (activated) on organ dysfunction in the PROWESS trial. Crit Care Med 2003; 31: 834–840.

40. Angus DC, Laterre PF, Helterbrand J, Ball D, Garg R, Bernard GR. The effects of drotrecogin alfa (activated) on long-term survival after sepsis [abstract]. Chest 2002; 122(Suppl): 51S.

41. Vincent JL, Levy MM, Macias WL, Trzaskoma BL. Early intervention with drotrecogin alfa (activated) improves survival benefit [abstract]. Crit Care Med 2003; 31: A123.

42. Bernard GR, Macias WL, Joyce DE, Williams MD, Bailey J, Vincent JL. Safety assessment of drotrecogin alfa (activated) in the treatment of adult patients with severe sepsis. Crit Care 2003; 7: 155–163.

43. Barton P, Kalil AC, Nadel S *et al.* Safety, pharmacokinetics, and pharmacodynamics of drotrecogin alfa (activated) in children with severe sepsis. Pediatrics 2004; 113: 7–17.
44. Van den Berghe G, Wouters P, Weekers F *et al.* Intensive insulin therapy in the critically ill patient. New Engl J Med 2001; 345: 1359–1367.
45. Annane D, Sebille V, Charpentier C *et al.* Effect of treatment with low doses of hydrocortisone and fludrocortisone on mortality in patients with septic shock. J Am Med Assoc 2002; 288: 862–871.
46. Manns BJ, Lee H, Doig CJ, Johnson D, Donaldson C. An economic evaluation of activated protein C treatment for severe sepsis. New Engl J Med 2002; 347: 993–1000.
47. Angus DC, Linde-Zwirble WT, Clermont G *et al.* Cost-effectiveness of drotrecogin alfa (activated) in the treatment of severe sepsis. Crit Care Med 2003; 31: 1–11.
48. Fowler RA, Hill-Popper M, Stasinos J, Petrou C, Sanders GD, Garber AM. Cost-effectiveness of recombinant human activated protein C and the influence of severity of illness in the treatment of patients with severe sepsis. J Crit Care 2003; 18: 181–191.
49. Betancourt M, McKinnon PS, Massanari RM, Kanji S, Bach D, Devlin JW. An evaluation of the cost effectiveness of drotrecogin alfa (activated) relative to the number of organ system failures. Pharmacoeconomics 2003; 21: 1331–1340.
50. Doig CJ, Zygun DA, Delaney A, Manns BJ. Drotrecogin alfa (activated; Xigris): and effective and cost-efficient treatment for severe sepsis. Expert Rev Pharmacoecon Outcome Res 2004; 4: 15–26.
51. Laterre PF, Heiselman D. Management of patients with severe sepsis, treated by drotrecogin alfa (activated). Am J Surg 2002; 184: S39–S46.
52. Levy MM, Fink MP, Marshall JC *et al.* 2001 SCCM/ESICM/ACCP/ATS/SIS International Sepsis Definitions Conference. Crit Care Med 2003; 31: 1250–1256.

H.K.F. van Saene   N. Taylor   S.P. Barrett
K. Lowry   R.E. Sarginson

Selective decontamination of the digestive tract: why don't we apply evidence in practice?

Introduction

Selective decontamination of the digestive tract (SDD) is a prophylactic strategy designed to prevent or minimize the impact of both endogenous and exogenous infections by potentially pathogenic micro-organisms (PPMs) in patients who require intensive care including mechanical ventilation. The purpose of SDD is to prevent or eradicate, if initially present, oropharyngeal and gastrointestinal carriage of PPMs, especially aerobic Gram-negative bacilli (AGNB), and also *Staphylococcus aureus* and yeasts, leaving the indigenous flora, which are thought to play a role in the resistance to colonization, predominantly undisturbed. The overall aim is a reduction in morbidity and mortality without antimicrobial resistance emerging.

Infection in the Intensive Care Unit

Morbidity and mortality due to infection, acquired either before or after admission to the intensive care unit (ICU), is a major problem in intensive care medicine.[1] The key to infection control in the ICU is to appreciate that a limited range of PPMs are involved and that infection with them usually follows a predictable endogenous pattern.[2] PPMs are first carried in the oropharynx and gut, before infection of internal organs such as lower airways and blood, develops. There are 15 common PPMs that cause practically all infections (Table 9.1). They can be classified into two groups: 'normal', usually carried by previously healthy people; and 'abnormal',

Table 9.1 PPMs causing infection during mechanical ventilation

Normal PPMs carried by previously **healthy individuals (%)**	
Streptococcus pneumoniae	60
Haemophilus influenzae	25–80
Moraxella catarrhalis	5
Escherichia coli	99
Candida albicans	30
Staphylococcus aureus (sensitive to methicillin)	30
Abnormal PPMs carried by **individuals with underlying disease**	
Klebsiella spp.	One-third when
Enterobacter spp.	APACHEII ⩾20
Citrobacter spp.	
Proteus spp.	
Morganella spp.	
Serratia spp.	
Acinetobacter spp.	
Pseudomonas spp.	
Staphylococcus aureus (resistant to methicillin)	

APACHE: Acute Physiologic and Chronic Health Evaluation.

usually harboured by individuals with a chronic or acute underlying condition. 'Normal' PPMs include *Streptococcus pneumoniae, Haemophilus influenzae, Moraxella catarrhalis, Escherichia coli, Staphylococcus aureus* and *Candida albicans*. The group of 'abnormal' bacteria causing infection on the ICU comprises eight AGNB and methicillin-resistant *Staphylococcus aureus* (MRSA). The AGNB are *Klebsiella, Enterobacter, Citrobacter, Proteus, Morganella, Acinetobacter, Serratia* and *Pseudomonas* species. Carriage of AGNB and MRSA in the oropharynx and gastrointestinal tract of healthy individuals is uncommon. Severity of illness is the most important factor in the conversion of the 'normal' into the 'abnormal' carrier state. In general, abnormal carriage develops early, within the first week of admission to the ICU, when the patient's illness is most severe and the associated immunodepression is maximal.

Exogenous infections should be distinguished from primary and secondary endogenous infections (Table 9.2). This classification is based on the carrier state of the ICU patient, which is only detectable using surveillance samples from throat and gut. Exogenous infections are less common (ca. 15%), but may occur throughout the patient's stay in the ICU, and are caused by 'abnormal' PPMs without previous carriage. For example, long-stay patients, particularly those who receive a tracheostomy, are at high risk of exogenous lower airway infections. Purulent lower airway secretions yield a PPM which has never been previously carried by the patient in the digestive tract flora or indeed in their oropharynx but has probably

Table 9.2 Three different types of ICU infection due to 15 PPMs

Type of infection	PPM	Carriage	Time cut-off	Incidence
Primary endogenous	Normal/abnormal	Present in admission flora	<1 week	ca. 55%
Secondary endogenous	Abnormal	Not present in admission flora, but acquired and carried later	>1 week	ca. 30%
Exogenous	Abnormal	No carriage at all	Any time throughout ICU treatment	ca. 15%

gained access via the tracheostomy. Causative bacteria are almost always abnormal AGNB such as *Acinetobacter* and *Pseudomonas* species, and MRSA. Both surveillance and diagnostic samples yield the same PPMs in infections of endogenous development. The most frequent infection in the ICU is primary endogenous infection caused by both 'normal' and 'abnormal' PPMs present in the admission flora (ca. 55%). Primary endogenous infections, in general, occur within the first week of admission to the ICU. If the patient was previously healthy (e.g. trauma and burn patients, patients with pancreatitis and acute liver failure), the bacteria causing early primary endogenous infections of lower airways and blood are usually the 'normal' PPMs. Abnormal MRSA and AGNB may cause primary endogenous infections, if the patient's defences are impaired by underlying disease. For example, a patient with chronic illness such as diabetes, alcoholism and chronic obstructive pulmonary disease may carry abnormal bacteria in the admission flora. Patients with debilitating conditions, transferred from other hospitals, wards or nursing homes, also have high abnormal carriage rates.

Secondary endogenous infections are invariably caused by 'abnormal' bacteria AGNB and MRSA that are within the ICU environment but are not present in the patient's admission flora. They are first acquired in the oropharynx followed by stomach and gut due to transmission via the hands of health care workers. In the critically ill patient, throat and gut acquisitions invariably lead to abnormal microbial carrier states, termed secondary or super carriage. The subsequent build-up to overgrowth, defined as 10^5 PPM/ml of saliva and/or g of faeces, may take a few days and can then result in colonization and subsequent secondary endogenous infection of lower airways and blood. One-third of ICU infections are secondary endogenous, and in general develop after 1 week of admission to the ICU.

What is SDD?

SDD is a prophylactic technique to control the three types of ICU infections due to the 15 PPMs.[3] The practice of SDD has four fundamental features (Table 9.3):

1. Enteral antimicrobials, applied in both the oropharynx and gut.

2. Parenteral antimicrobials given immediately on admission.

3. Hand hygiene.

4. Surveillance cultures of throat and rectum.

This strategy selectively targets the 15 PPMs which contribute to morbidity and mortality. By design SDD does not target low-level pathogens including anaerobes, viridans streptococci, enterococci and coagulase-negative staphylococci as, in general, they only cause morbidity. The most important feature of SDD is the enteral administration of oral non-absorbable polymyxin E/tobramycin to eradicate the abnormal AGNB. This results in decontamination of the digestive tract. SDD is a manoeuvre designed to convert the 'abnormal' carrier state into the 'normal' carrier state using

Table 9.3 Full four component protocol of SDD

Target PPM and antimicrobials	Total daily dose (4 × daily)		
	<5 years	5–12 years	>12 years
Enteral antimicrobials			
Oropharynx			
• AGNB: polymyxin E with tobramycin		2 g of 2% paste or gel	
• Yeasts: amphotericin B or nystatin		2 g of 2% paste or gel	
• MRSA: vancomycin		2 g of 4% paste or gel	
Gut			
• AGNB: polymyxin E (mg) with	100	200	400
tobramycin (mg)	80	160	320
• Yeasts: amphotericin B (mg) or	500	1000	2000
nystatin (units)	2×10^6	4×10^6	8×10^6
• MRSA: vancomycin (mg)	20–40/kg	20–40/kg	500–2000
Parenteral antimicrobials			
Cefotaxime (mg)	150/kg	200/kg	4000
Hygiene			
Surveillance cultures of throat and rectum On admission, Monday, Thursday			

non-absorbable enteral antimicrobials. Critically ill patients are unable to clear these AGNB due to their underlying disease. Intestinal overgrowth with AGNB causes systemic immunoparalysis. The reasons for the administration of enteral polymyxin E/tobramycin is that it provides recovery of systemic immunity, and that prevention or eradication of abnormal AGNB in throat and gut effectively controls aspiration and translocation of these micro-organisms into the lower airways and blood, respectively. Enteral antimicrobials have been shown to be effective in the control of *secondary endogenous* infections. However, the use of enteral antibiotics alone does not affect primary endogenous and exogenous infections. The second component is the immediate administration of an adequate parenteral antimicrobial to control *primary endogenous* pneumonia and septicaemia. Cefotaxime has been used in most randomized controlled trials (RCTs) to cover both 'normal' and 'abnormal' PPMs. In adding enteral to parenteral antibiotics, the original pre-1980s systemic antibiotics, including cefotaxime, remain useful, without the development of antimicrobial resistance. Thirdly, high standards of hygiene are indispensable for reducing hand contamination and subsequent transmission from '*external*' sources. Finally, surveillance samples of throat and rectum, unpopular among traditional microbiologists, are taken on admission and twice weekly thereafter, and are an integral component of the SDD protocol. Knowledge of the carrier state allows the compliance and efficacy of this prophylactic protocol to be monitored.

What is the Evidence?

Fifty-four RCTs[4–57] were designed to evaluate SDD in a total of 8715 patients between 1987 and 2004, and there are seven meta-analyses of the RCTs assessing SDD.[58–64] Thirty-eight RCTs show a significant reduction in infection and four in mortality. All meta-analyses show a significant reduction in infection and five out of seven meta-analyses report a significant mortality reduction. The most recent meta-analysis includes 36 RCTs in 6922 patients, and shows that SDD reduces the odds ratio for pneumonia to 0.35 (95% confidence interval (CI) 0.29–0.41), and mortality to 0.78 (95% CI 0.68–0.89).[64] Five ICU patients need to be treated with SDD to prevent one pneumonia, and 21 ICU patients need to be treated to prevent one death. Two recent large RCTs[26,29] report an absolute mortality reduction of 8% corresponding to the treatment of 12 patients with SDD to save one life.

Antimicrobial resistance among AGNB has never been a problem over a period of 17 years of clinical ICU research. Five SDD studies prospectively evaluated resistance for 2, 2.5, 4, 6 and 7 years.[65–69] No increase in the

Table 9.4 ICU interventions that reduce mortality

Intervention	Relative risk (95% CI)	Absolute mort reduction (%) (95% CI)	Number needed to treat
Low tidal volume	0.78 (0.65–0.93)	8.8 (2.4–15.3)	11
Activated protein C	0.80 (0.69–0.94)	6.1 (1.9–10.4)	16
Intensive insulin	0.44 (0.36–0.81)	3.7 (1.3–6.1)	27
>5 days	0.52 (0.33–0.84)	9.6 (3.0–16.1)	10
Steroids	0.90 (0.74–1.09)	6.4 (−4.8–17.6)	16
Non-responders to 0.25 mg of tetracosactrin	0.83 (0.66–1.04)	10.8 (−1.9–23.6)	9
Selective decontamination	0.65 (0.49–0.85)	8.1 (3.1–13.0)	12

rate of superinfections due to resistant AGNB could be demonstrated. The latest RCT, evaluating SDD in about 1000 patients, had significantly fewer carriers of multi-resistant AGNB in the patients receiving SDD than in the control group.[26] Six RCTs, conducted in ICUs where MRSA was endemic at the time of the study, showed a trend towards higher MRSA infection rates in patients receiving SDD.[17,20,23,31,53,54] Under these circumstances, SDD requires the addition of oropharyngeal and enteral vancomycin. Four studies, two of which were RCTs, support the method of surveillance cultures combined with enteral vancomycin.[70–73] The carriage and infection rates of vancomycin-resistant enterococci were low and similar in test and control group.[6,24,57,71] Recent literature shows that parenteral antibiotics that do not respect the patient's gut ecology rather than high doses of enteral vancomycin, promote the emergence of vancomycin-resistant enterococci in the gut.[74,75]

The most recent data showing a survival benefit without bacterial resistance emerging support level 1 evidence for SDD, allowing a grade A recommendation. Table 9.4 shows the five evidence-based medicine (EBM) manoeuvres showing survival benefit in the critically ill. Only SDD is supported by at least two level 1 investigations,[26,29] the other four[76–79] are supported by only one trial, providing a grade B recommendation. In addition, SDD can be administered to all patients at risk of infection, while the other four only in specific subsets of critically ill patients.

Why is SDD not Widely Used?

Two recent surveys into the usage of SDD reveal that it is routinely used in only 4% of UK ICUs,[80] but in 24% of Dutch ICUs.[81] The most common reason cited for its non-use (83%) is the belief by UK intensivists that there is a lack of evidence of efficacy and 'it does not work'.[80] The reason for this misconception is multifactorial. However, the longstanding disagreement among experts[82,83] has been an important factor contributing to the confusion. History repeats itself in that Semmelweis' work was heavily opposed by Virchow, the expert pathologist of that time.[84]

The main reason for SDD not being widely used is the primacy of opinion over evidence. Previous experience with thrombolytic drugs indicates a similar pattern, with an undesirable lag between the appearance of meta-analytic evidence and the recommendations of experts. Streptokinase was shown to reduce the risk of death from myocardial infarction by 20% as long ago as 1975. During the following two decades 14 review articles either failed to mention streptokinase or considered it still to be experimental,[85] although in this century streptokinase is virtually routine treatment in patients with myocardial infarction.

Concerns expressed about resistance have also hindered the implementation of SDD. All analyses of antimicrobial resistance associated with SDD[83,86–89] are based on case reports and review articles rather than evidence. A statement based on expert opinion is misleading and runs contrary to the aims of EBM – the best estimate based on an impartial review of all available information. Among other concerns, the denominator in many reviews is isolates, samples or infections, not patients.[53,86] All reviews include the six RCTs which were conducted in ICUs where MRSA was endemic at the time of the trial, although there was only a trend towards a higher MRSA infection rate in the patients receiving SDD.[17,20,23,31,53,54] A statistically significant trend towards resistance among Gram-positive bacteria was found only if including rates of carriage and infection due to low-level pathogens such as enterococci and coagulase-negative staphylococci. Clearly, pneumonia due to these low-level pathogens is extremely rare. Finally, exogenous infections are not controlled by SDD. A transient increase in exogenous lower airway infections due to *Acinetobacter baumannii* was reported from a respiratory unit with a high percentage of tracheotomized patients while conducting a RCT on SDD.[65] This observation that the proportion of exogenous infections in SDD trials increases in relation to the reduction in endogenous infections is well recognized. This transient finding is repeatedly used to show that SDD increases resistance among AGNB.[89] The assertion that resistance is a problem with SDD is misplaced in an evidence-based analysis.

Since its inception, SDD has rarely received a favourable press.[83,86–89] Indeed, the 1992 report[90] of the *First European Consensus Conference* in Paris, France set the scene by coming down against the use of SDD. In the same vein, although SDD has been a regular feature on the programme of the *Annual Intensive Care* meeting in Brussels, Belgium, since 1987, in only three years (1988, 1990, 2003) were speakers invited who viewed it in a favourable light. A greater acceptability for publication of manuscripts that show negative results for SDD compounds its poor reputation – of the 54 randomized trials of SDD, the six showing no benefit[17,20,23,31,53,54] were all published by journals of high impact factor. An extreme example is the publication by the *New England Journal of Medicine* of an uncontrolled study where 10% of the study population developed enterococcal pneumonia.[91] It might be questioned whether such a high incidence of such an obscure condition should be taken at face value.

SDD has also never been promoted by pharmaceutical companies, perhaps because there is little profit in older agents such as cefotaxime, polymyxin E, tobramycin and amphotericin B, which are inexpensive and off-patent. Furthermore, SDD is not supported by authoritative-looking data sheets and is not marketed to clinicians in the traditional manner. Paste, gel and suspension are not readily available on the shelf. Hence, the application of SDD requires more effort in terms of commitment and monitoring from the ICU team than is the case with mere systemic administration of the latest antibiotic on the market.

Finally, Wazana questions the interaction of physicians and the pharmaceutical industry and asks 'Is a gift ever just a gift?'.[92] Most opinion leaders have links with the industry and receive grants for the evaluation of new antimicrobial agents both *in vitro* and *in vivo*. The same experts attend national and international meetings at which they chair and report data often promoting these new drugs as first-line antibiotics. The traditionalists on the 'circuit' have relied on the industry to develop new drugs at regular intervals, usually 2 years following publication of the first case report of superinfections of the currently favoured antibiotic. The realization that the pharmaceutical industry failed to provide new classes of antibiotics came as a severe blow. Industrialized countries have largely delegated control of drug trials to pharmaceutical companies,[93] which places clear limitations on research. However, economic interests seek the best possible financial return, and establishing new potent antibiotics to treat rather than prevent pneumonia is more profitable. Antibiotic usage in the (UK) National Health Service is mainly determined by the pharmaceutical industry. The replacement of piperacillin by piperacillin/tazobactam illustrates that the importance of market forces and financial incentives is placed far above public health needs.

The Future

In spite of the powerful anti-SDD movement, SDD is now an EBM protocol. Influential European,[94] UK[95] and US[96] societies and institutions acknowledge that SDD is the best-ever evaluated intervention in intensive care medicine that reduces infectious morbidity and mortality. The US Department for Health and Human Services considers SDD to be a cheap manoeuvre.[96]

Perhaps the most intriguing aspect of the 17 years of clinical research into SDD is the experience that the addition of enteral antibiotics to parenteral antimicrobials may prolong the antibiotic era. Pre-1980s antibiotics are still active so long as they are combined with eradication of AGNB and MRSA from the gut. We believe that the answer lies not in the development of single, new, more potent and expensive systemic antimicrobials but in a radical re-thinking of the philosophy by which antimicrobials are used. In particular, we need to be much more critical of market-driven health care if we are to find more sustainable solutions to the problems of the ongoing spread of nosocomial, antibiotic-resistant pathogens in the new millennium.

References

1. Angus DC, Linde-Zwirble WT, Lidicker J et al. Epidemiology of severe sepsis in the United States: analysis of incidence, outcome and associated costs of care. Crit Care Med 2001; 29: 1303–1310.
2. Baxby D, van Saene HKF, Stoutenbeek CP, Zandstra DF. Selective decontamination of the digestive tract: 13 years on, what it is and what it is not. Intens Care Med 1996; 22: 699–706.
3. van Saene HKF, Petros AJ, Ramsay G, Baxby D. All great truths are iconoclastic: selective decontamination of the digestive tract moves from heresy to level 1 truth. Intens Care Med 2003; 29: 677–690.
4. Abele-Horn M, Dauber A, Bauernfeind A, Russwurm W, Seyfarth-Metzger I, Gleich P et al. Decrease in nosocomial pneumonia in ventilated patients by selective oropharyngeal decontamination (SOD). Intens Care Med 1997; 23: 187–195.
5. Aerdts SJ, van Dalen R, Clasener HA, Festen J, van Lier HJ, Vollaard EJ. Antibiotic prophylaxis of respiratory tract infection in mechanically ventilated patients. A prospective, blinded, randomized trial of the effect of a novel regimen. Chest 1991; 100: 783–791.
6. Arnow PM, Carandang GC, Zabner R, Irwin ME. Randomized controlled trial of selective bowel decontamination for prevention of infections following liver transplantation. Clin Infect Dis 1996; 22: 997–1003.
7. Barret JP, Jeschke MG, Herndon DN. Selective decontamination of the digestive tract in severely burned pediatric patients. Burns 2001; 27: 439–445.
8. Bergmans DC, Bonten MJ, Gaillard CA, Paling JC, van der Geest S, van Tiel FH et al. Prevention of ventilator-associated pneumonia by oral decontamination: a prospective, randomized, double-blind, placebo-controlled study. Am J Respir Crit Care Med 2001; 164: 382–388.
9. Bion JF, Badger I, Crosby HA, Hutchings P, Kong KL, Baker J et al. Selective decontamination of the digestive tract reduces Gram-negative pulmonary colonization but not systemic endotoxemia in patients undergoing elective liver transplantation. Crit Care Med 1994; 22: 40–49.

10. Blair P, Rowlands BJ, Lowry K, Webb H, Armstrong P, Smilie J. Selective decontamination of the digestive tract: a stratified, randomized, prospective study in a mixed intensive care unit. Surgery 1991; 110: 303–309.

11. Boland JP, Sadler DL, Stewart W, Wood DJ, Zerick W, Snodgras KR. Reduction of nosocomial respiratory infections in multiple trauma patients requiring mechanical ventilation by selective parenteral and enteral antisepsis regimen (SPEAR) in the intensive care. Seventeenth International Congress of Chemotherapy Berlin 1991; Abstract No. 0465.

12. Bouter H, Schippers EF, Luelmo SA, Versteegh MI, Ros P, Guiot HF et al. No effect of preoperative selective gut decontamination on endotoxemia and cytokine activation during cardiopulmonary bypass: a randomized, placebo-controlled study. Crit Care Med 2002; 30: 38–43.

13. Brun-Buisson C, Legrand P, Rauss A, Montravers F, Besbes M, Meakins JL et al. Intestinal decontamination for control of nosocomial multi-resistant Gram-negative bacilli. Ann Intern Med 1989; 110: 873–881.

14. de la Cal MA, Cerda E, Garcia-Hierro P et al. Survival benefit in severely burned patients receiving selective decontamination of the digestive tract: a randomized, double blind, placebo controlled trial. Med Intens 2002; 26: 152: Abstract 028.

15. Cerra FB, Maddaus MA, Dunn DL, Wells CL, Konstantinides NN, Lehman SL et al. Selective gut decontamination reduces nosocomial infections and length of stay but not mortality or organ failure in surgical intensive care unit patients. Arch Surg 1992; 127: 163–169.

16. Cockerill III FR, Muller SR, Anhalt JP, Marsh HM, Farnell MB, Mucha P et al. Prevention of infection in critically ill patients by selective decontamination of the digestive tract. Ann Intern Med 1992; 117: 545–553.

17. Ferrer M, Torres A, Gonzalez J, de la Bellacasa JP, El-Ebiary M, Roca M. Utility of selective digestive decontamination in mechanically ventilated patients. Ann Intern Med 1994; 120: 389–395.

18. Finch RG, Tomlinson P, Holliday M, Sole K, Stack C, Rocker G. Selective decontamination of the digestive tract (SDD) in the prevention of secondary sepsis in a medical/surgical intensive care unit. Seventeenth International Congress of Chemotherapy Berlin 1991; Abstract No. 0471.

19. Flaherty J, Nathan C, Kabins SA, Weinstein RA. Pilot trial of selective decontamination for prevention of bacterial infection in an intensive care unit. J Infect Dis 1990; 162: 1393–1397.

20. Gastinne H, Wolff M, Delatour F, Faurisson F, Chevret S. A controlled trial in intensive care units of selective decontamination of the digestive tract with non-absorbable antibiotics. New Engl J Med 1992; 326: 594–599.

21. Gaussorgues P, Salord F, Sirodot M, Tigaud S, Cagnin S, Gerard M et al. Efficacité de la décontamination digestive sur la survenue des bactériémies nosocomiales chez les patients sous ventilation méchanique et recevant des betamimétiques. Réanimation Soins Intensifs Médecin d'Urgence 1991; 7: 169–174.

22. Georges B, Mazerolles M, Decun J-F, Rouge P, Pomies S, Cougot P et al. Décontamination digestive sélective résultats d'une étude chez polytraumatisés. Réanimation Urgence 1994; 3: 621–627.

23. Hammond JM, Potgieter PD, Saunders GL, Forder AA. Double-blind study of selective decontamination of the digestive tract in intensive care. Lancet 1992; 340: 5–9.

24. Hellinger WC, Yao JD, Alvarez S, Blair JE, Cawley JJ, Paya CV *et al.* A randomized, prospective, double-blinded evaluation of selective bowel decontamination in liver transplantation. Transplantation 2002; 73: 1904–1909.

25. Jacobs S, Foweraker JE, Roberts SE. Effectiveness of selective decontamination of the digestive tract (SDD) in an ICU with a policy encouraging a low gastric pH. Clin Intens Care 1992; 3: 52–58.

26. de Jonge E, Schultz MJ, Spanjaard L, Bossuyt PMM, Vroom MB, Dankert J *et al.* Effects of selective decontamination of digestive tract on mortality and acquisition of resistant bacteria in intensive care: a randomised controlled trial. Lancet 2003; 362: 1011–1016.

27. Kerver AJH, Rommes JH, Mevissen-Verhage EAE, Hulstaert PF, Vos A, Verhoef J *et al.* Prevention of colonization and infection in critically ill patients: a prospective randomized study. Crit Care Med 1988; 16: 1087–1093.

28. Korinek AM, Laisne MJ, Nicolas MH, Raskine L, Deroin V, Sanson-Lepors MJ. Selective decontamination of the digestive tract in neurosurgical intensive care unit patients: a double-blind, randomized, placebo-controlled study. Crit Care Med 1993; 21: 1466–1473.

29. Krueger WA, Lenhart FP, Neeser G, Ruckdeschel G, Schreckhase H, Eissner HJ *et al.* Influence of combined intravenous and topical antibiotic prophylaxis on the incidence of infections, organ dysfunctions, and mortality in critically ill surgical patients: a prospective, stratified, randomized, double-blind, placebo-controlled clinical trial. Am J Respir Crit Care Med 2002; 166: 1029–1037.

30. Laggner AN, Tryba M, Georgopoulos A, Lenz K, Grimm G, Graninger W *et al.* Oropharyngeal decontamination with gentamicin for long-term ventilated patients on stress ulcer prophylaxis with sucralfate? Wien Klin Wochenschr 1994; 106: 15–19.

31. Lingnau W, Berger J, Javorsky F, Lejeune P, Mutz N, Benzer H. Selective intestinal decontamination in multiple trauma patients: prospective, controlled trial. J Trauma 1997; 42: 687–694.

32. Luiten EJT, Hop WCJ, Lange JF, Bruining HA. Controlled clinical trial of selective decontamination for the treatment of severe acute pancreatitis. Ann Surg 1995; 222: 57–65.

33. Martinez-Pellus AE, Merino P, Bru M, Conejero R, Seller G, Munoz C *et al.* Can selective digestive decontamination avoid the endotoxemia and cytokine activation promoted by cardiopulmonary bypass? Crit Care Med 1993; 21: 1684–1691.

34. Martinez-Pellus AE, Merino P, Bru M, Canovas J, Seller G, Sapina J *et al.* Endogenous endotoxemia of intestinal origin during cardiopulmonary bypass. Role of type of flow and protective effect of selective digestive decontamination. Intens Care Med 1997; 23: 1251–1257.

35. Palomar M, Alvarez-Lerma F, Jorda R, Bermejo B, for the Catalan Study Group of Nosocomial Pneumonia Prevention. Prevention of nosocomial pneumonia in mechanically ventilated patients: selective decontamination versus sucralfate. Clin Intens Care 1997; 8: 228–235.

36. Pneumatikos I, Koulouras V, Nathanail C, Goe D, Nakos G. Selective decontamination of subglottic area in mechanically ventilated patients with multiple trauma. Intens Care Med 2002; 28: 432–437.

37. Pugin J, Auckenthaler R, Lew DP, Suter PM. Oropharyngeal decontamination decreases incidence of ventilator-associated pneumonia. A randomized, placebo-controlled, double-blind clinical trial. J Am Med Assoc 1991; 265: 2704–2710.

38. Quinio B, Albanese J, Bues-Charbit M, Viviand X, Martin C. Selective decontamination of the digestive tract in multiple trauma patients. A prospective, double-blind, randomized, placebo-controlled study. Chest 1996; 109: 765–772.

39. Rayes N, Seehofer D, Hansen S et al. Early enteral supply of *Lactobacillus* and fibre versus selective bowel decontamination: A controlled trial in liver transplant recipients. Transplantation 2002; 74: 123–128.

40. Rocha LA, Martin MJ, Pita S, Paz J, Seco C, Margusino L et al. Prevention of nosocomial infections in critically ill patients by selective decontamination of the digestive tract. A randomised, double blind, placebo controlled study. Intens Care Med 1992; 18: 398–404.

41. Rodriguez-Roldan JM, Altuna-Cuesta A, Lopez A, Carrillo A, Garcia J, Leon J et al. Prevention of nosocomial lung infection in ventilated patients: use of an antimicrobial pharyngeal nonabsorbable paste. Crit Care Med 1990; 18: 1239–1242.

42. Rolando N, Gimson A, Wade J, Philpott-Howard J, Casewell M, Williams R. Prospective controlled trial of selective parenteral and enteral antimicrobial regimen in fulminant liver failure. Hepatology 1993; 17: 196–201.

43. Rolando N, Wade JJ, Stangou A, Gimson AE, Wendon J, Philpott-Howard J et al. Prospective study comparing the efficacy of prophylactic parenteral antimicrobials, with or without enteral decontamination, in patients with acute liver failure. Liver Transpl Surg 1996; 2: 8–13.

44. Ruza F, Alvarado F, Herruzo R, Delgado MA, Garcia S, Dorao P et al. Prevention of nosocomial infection in a pediatric intensive care unit (PICU) through the use of selective digestive decontamination. Eur J Epidemiol 1998; 14: 719–727.

45. Sanchez GM, Cambronero Galache JA, Lopez DJ, Cerda CE, Rubio BJ, Gomez Aguinaga MA et al. Effectiveness and cost of selective decontamination of the digestive tract in critically ill intubated patients. A randomized, double-blind, placebo-controlled, multicenter trial. Am J Respir Crit Care Med 1998; 158: 908–916.

46. Schardey HM, Joosten U, Finke U, Staubach KH, Schauer R, Heiss A et al. The prevention of anastomotic leakage after total gastrectomy with local decontamination. A prospective, randomized, double-blind, placebo-controlled multicenter trial. Ann Surg 1997; 225: 172–180.

47. Smith SD, Jackson RJ, Hannakan CJ, Wadowsky RM, Tzakis AG, Rowe MI. Selective decontamination in pediatric liver transplants. A randomized prospective study. Transplantation 1993; 55: 1306–1309.

48. Stoutenbeek CP, van Saene HKF, Zandstra DF. Prevention of multiple organ system failure by selective decontamination of the digestive tract in multiple trauma patients. In: Faist EBAE, Schildberg FW (eds) Immune Consequences of Trauma, Shock and Sepsis. Lengerich: Pabst Science Publishers, 1996; 1055–1066.

49. Stoutenbeek CP, van Saene II, Little RA, Whitehead A. The effect of selective decontamination of the digestive tract on mortality in multiple trauma patients. J Trauma 2004; submitted.

50. Tetteroo GW, Wagenvoort JH, Castelein A, Tilanus HW, Ince C, Bruining HA. Selective decontamination to reduce Gram-negative colonisation and infections after oesophageal resection. Lancet 1990; 335: 704–707.

51. Ulrich C, Harinck-de Weerd JE, Bakker NC, Jacz K, Doornbos L, de Ridder VA. Selective decontamination of the digestive tract with norfloxacin in the

prevention of ICU-acquired infections: a prospective, randomized study. Intens Care Med 1989; 15: 424–431.

52. Unertl K, Ruckdeschel G, Selbmann HK, Jensen U, Forst H, Lenhart FP *et al.* Prevention of colonization and respiratory infections in long-term ventilated patients by local antimicrobial prophylaxis. Intens Care Med 1987; 13: 106–113.

53. Verwaest C, Verhaegen J, Ferdinande P, Schets M, Berghe vd G, Verbist L. Randomized controlled trial of selective digestive decontamination in 600 mechanically ventilated patients in a multi-disciplinary intensive care unit. Crit Care Med 1997; 25: 63–71.

54. Wiener J, Itokazu G, Nathan C, Kabins SA, Weinstein RA. A randomized, double-blind, placebo controlled trial of selective digestive decontamination in a medical, surgical intensive care unit. Clin Infect Dis 1995; 20: 861–867.

55. Winter R, Humphreys H, Pick A, MacGowan AP, Willatts SM, Speller DC. A controlled trial of selective decontamination of the digestive tract in intensive care and its effect on nosocomial infection. J Antimicrob Chemother 1992; 30: 73–87.

56. Zobel G, Kuttnig M, Grubbauer HM, Semmelrock HJ, Thiel W. Reduction of colonization and infection rate during pediatric intensive care by selective decontamination of the digestive tract. Crit Care Med 1991; 19: 1242–1246.

57. Zwaveling JH, Maring JK, Klompmaker IJ, Haagsma EB, Bottema JT, Laseur M *et al.* Selective decontamination of the digestive tract to prevent postoperative infection: a randomized placebo-controlled trial in liver transplant patients. Crit Care Med 2002; 30: 1204–1209.

58. Selective Decontamination of the Digestive Tract Trialists Collaborative Group. Meta-analysis of randomised controlled trials of selective decontamination of the digestive tract. Br Med J 1993; 307: 525–532.

59. Heyland DK, Cook DJ, Jaescher R, Griffith L, Lee HN, Guyatt GH. Selective decontamination of the digestive tract. An overview. Chest 1994; 105: 1221–1229.

60. Kollef M. The role of selective digestive tract decontamination on mortality and respiratory tract infections. Chest 1994; 105: 1101–1108.

61. D'Amico R, Pifferi S, Leonetti C, Torri V, Tinazzi A, Liberati A. Effectiveness of antibiotic prophylaxis in critically ill adult patients: systematic review of randomized controlled trials. Br Med J 1998; 316:1275–1285.

62. Nathens AB, Marshall JC. Selective decontamination of the digestive tract in surgical patients. A systematic review of the evidence. Arch Surg 1999; 134: 170–176.

63. Redman R, Ludington E, Crocker M, Wittes J, Bellm J, Carlet J and the VAP advisory group. Analysis of respiratory and non-respiratory infections in published trials of selective decontamination. Intens Care Med 2001; 27(Suppl): Abstract No. 586: S285.

64. Liberati A, D'Amico R, Pifferi S *et al.* Antibiotic prophylaxis to reduce respiratory tract infections and mortality in adults receiving intensive care. Cochrane Review, The Cochrane Library, Issue 1. Chichester, UK: John Wiley & Sons Ltd., 2004.

65. Hammond JMJ, Potgieter PD. Long-term effects of selective decontamination on antimicrobial resistance. Crit Care Med 1995; 23: 637–645.

66. Stoutenbeek CP, van Saene HKF, Zandstra DF. The effect of oral non-absorbable antibiotics on the emergence of resistant bacteria in patients in an intensive care unit. J Antimicrob Chemother 1987; 19: 513–520.

67. Lingnau W, Berger J, Javorsky F *et al.* Changing bacterial ecology during a five year period of selective intestinal decontamination. J Hosp Infect 1998; 39: 195–206.

68. Leone M, Albanese J, Antonini F *et al.* Long-term (6-year) effect of selective decontamination on antimicrobial resistance in intensive care, multiple-trauma patients. Crit Care Med 2003; 31: 2090–2095.

69. Tetteroo GWM, Wagenvoort JHT, Bruining HA. Bacteriology of selective decontamination: efficacy and rebound colonization. J Antimicrob Chemother 1994; 34: 139–148.

70. Silvestri L, Milanese M, Oblach L *et al.* Enteral vancomycin to control methicillin-resistant *Staphylococcus aureus* outbreak in mechanically ventilated patients. Am J Infect Cont 2002; 30: 391–399.

71. de la Cal MA, Cerda E, van Saene HKF *et al.* Effectiveness and safety of enteral vancomycin to control endemicity of methicillin-resistant *Staphylococcus aureus* in a medical/surgical intensive care unit. J Hosp Infect 2004; 56: 175–183.

72. Silvestri L, van Saene HKF, Milanese M *et al.* Prevention of MRSA pneumonia by oral vancomycin decontamination: a randomized trial. Eur Respir J 2004; 23: 921–926.

73. Sanchez M, Mir N, Canton R *et al.* The effect of topical vancomycin on acquisition, carriage and infection with methicillin-resistant *Staphylococcus aureus* in critically ill patients. A double-blind, randomized, placebo-controlled study. 37th ICAAC, Toronto, Canada 1997; Abstract No. J-119, p. 310.

74. Stiefel U, Paterson DL, Pultz NJ *et al.* Effect of increasing use of piperacillin/tazobactam on the incidence of vancomycin-resistant enterococci in four academic medical centers. Infect Cont Hosp Epidemiol 2004; 25: 380–383.

75. Salgado CD, Giannetta ET, Farr BM. Failure to develop vancomycin-resistant *Enterococcus* with oral vancomycin treatment of *Clostridium difficile*. Infect Cont Hosp Epidemiol 2004; 25: 413–417.

76. The Acute Respiratory Distress Syndrome Network. Ventilation with lower tidal volumes as compared with traditional tidal volumes for acute lung injury and the acute respiratory distress syndrome. New Engl J Med 2000; 342: 1301–1308.

77. Bernard GR, Vincent J-L, Laterre PF *et al.* Efficacy and safety of recombinant human activated protein C for severe sepsis. New Engl J Med 2001; 344: 699–709.

78. van den Berghe G, Wouters P, Weekers F *et al.* Intensive insulin therapy in critically ill patients. New Engl J Med 2001; 245: 1359–1367.

79. Annane D, Sebille V, Charpentier C *et al.* Effect of treatment with low doses of hydrocortisone and fluorocortisone on mortality in patient with septic shock. J Am Med Assoc 2002; 288: 862–871.

80. Nixon JR, Nielsen MS. Selective decontamination of the digestive tract – current national practice. Br J Anaesth 2000; 84: 682P–683P.

81. Bogaards MJ. An inventarisation of the products. Selective digestive decontamination in the Netherlands. Pharm Weekblad 2001; 136: 706–712.

82. Aarts MA, Marshall JC. In defense of evidence. The continuing saga of selective decontamination of the digestive tract. Am J Respir Crit Care Med 2002; 166: 1014–1015.

83. Vincent JL. Selective digestive decontamination for everyone, everywhere? Lancet 2003; 362: 1006–1007.

84. Farr BM. Reasons for non-compliance with infection control guidelines. Infect Cont Hosp Epidemiol 2000; 21: 411–416.

85. Antman EM, Lau J, Kupelnick B *et al*. A comparison of results of meta-analyses of randomized control trials and recommendation of clinical experts. J Am Med Assoc 1992; 268: 240–248.
86. Nardi G, Valentinis U, Proietti A *et al*. Epidemiological impact of prolonged systemic use of topical SDD on bacterial colonization of the tracheo-bronchial tree and antibiotic resistance. Intens Care Med 1993; 19: 273–278.
87. Ebner W, Kropec-Hubner A, Daschner FD. Bacterial resistance and overgrowth due to selective decontamination of the digestive tract. Eur J Clin Microbiol Infect Dis 2000; 19: 243–247.
88. Collard HR, Saint S, Matthay MA. Prevention of ventilator-associated pneumonia. Comments and responses. Ann Intern Med 2004; 140: 486–487.
89. Kollef MH. Selective digestive decontamination should not be routinely employed. Chest 2003; 123: 464S–468S.
90. European Society of Intensive Care Medicine, Société Réanimation de Langue Française. The First European Consensus Conference in Intensive Care Medicine: selective decontamination of the digestive tract in intensive care patients. Infect Cont Hosp Epidemiol 1992; 13: 609–611.
91. Bonten MJM, van Tiel FH, van der Geest S *et al*. *Enterococcus faecalis* pneumonia complicating topical antimicrobial prophylaxis. New Engl J Med 1993; 328: 209–210.
92. Wazana A. Physicians and the pharmaceutical industry. Is a gift ever just a gift? J Am Med Assoc 2000; 283: 373–380.
93. Garattini S, Liberati A. The risk of bias from omitted research. Evidence must be independently sought and free of economic interests. Br Med J 2000; 321: 845–846.
94. Torres A, Carlet J, European Task Force on Ventilator-Associated Pneumonia. Ventilator-associated pneumonia. Eur Respir J 2001; 17: 1034–1045.
95. Royal College of Pathologists. Continuing professional development. J Hosp Infect 2002; 50: 161.
96. University of California at San Francisco, Stanford University Evidence-Based Practice Center. Making health care safer: a critical analysis of patient safety practice. www.ahrg.gov/clinic/ptsafety 2001.

D. Mesotten   I. Vanhorebeek   G. Van den Berghe

Glycaemic control and outcome in intensive care

When Banting and Best discovered insulin in 1922, it was a revolutionary breakthrough, since it became possible to treat patients with Type 1 diabetes mellitus, a disorder that had previously been lethal due to the development of ketoacidosis. At the end of the 19th century, Claude Bernard described that acute trauma was associated with the development of hyperglycaemia. The rise in blood glucose levels was considered to be an adaptive stress response and proceeded irrespective of underlying diabetes. Since then, it has become clear that hyperglycaemia also commonly develops during other types of critical illness besides trauma. Conventionally, hyperglycaemia in critical illness was only treated when blood glucose levels became excessively elevated. However, a recent study has clearly established the beneficial effects of treating even moderate hyperglycaemia in critically ill patients.[1]

Altered Glucose Regulation in Trauma and Critical Illness

The concept 'stress diabetes' or 'diabetes of injury' has been in the literature for almost 150 years. The stress imposed by severe trauma, burns and critical illness leads to the development of hyperglycaemia as a result of the integrated action of hormonal, cytokine and nervous 'counter-regulatory' signals on glucose metabolic pathways. In the acute stage of the disease, hepatic glucose synthesis is enhanced in the critically ill patient by both increased gluconeogenesis and glycogenolysis. Hepatic gluconeogenesis is assumed to be upregulated by increased levels of glucagon, cortisol and growth hormone.[2,3] The catecholamines adrenaline and noradrenaline, which are released in response to acute injury, stimulate hepatic glycogenolysis.[4] Moreover, several cytokines, including interleukin-1,[5,6] interleukin-6 and tumour necrosis factor[7] may directly or indirectly enhance both these hyperglycaemic responses. The evolution of intensive care medicine during the last three to four decades has fostered a dramatic increase in the survival of patients under conditions of multiple trauma, extensive burns and severe sepsis, among others. Hence, patients now frequently enter the chronic phase of critical illness.[8] The mechanisms regulating hyperglycaemia during protracted critical illness remain relatively unclear. In the acute phase, concentrations of growth hormone, cortisol, catecholamine and cytokines are usually lower than in the more chronic phase of critical illness, but the change in glucagon concentration is not well documented.[9,10] Apart from the higher rate of glucose production, the glucose uptake mechanisms are also affected during critical illness. First of all, the immobilization of the patient results in the almost total disappearance of the important exercise-stimulated glucose uptake in skeletal muscle. Furthermore, the insulin-stimulated glucose uptake is compromised due to a combined inhibition of insulin-stimulated glucose uptake by glucose transporter-4 (GLUT-4) as well as glycogen synthase.[11,12] The data reported on glucose oxidation through pyruvate produced in the glycolytic pathway are controversial, some studies showed decreased oxidation rates,[13] whereas the opposite effect has been demonstrated by others.[14] However, the decrease in insulin-stimulated glucose uptake in skeletal muscle and adipose tissue is completely compensated for by a massive increase in total body glucose uptake, of which the mononuclear phagocyte system in liver, spleen and ileum is the main receiver.[15] The overall increased peripheral glucose uptake[16] in view of hyperglycaemia only underscores the pivotal role of the rise in hepatic glucose production during critical illness, which cannot be suppressed by exogenous glucose.[17] The hepatic synthesis of glucose by gluconeogenesis and glycogenolysis is normally inhibited by insulin. The combined picture of higher serum insulin levels, impaired peripheral glucose uptake and elevated hepatic glucose production points to the development of insulin resistance during critical illness.

Historical Rationale for the Management of Hyperglycaemia in Critical Care

Normally, blood glucose levels are tightly regulated within the narrow range of 3.3–7.7 mmol/l (60–140 mg/dl) both in fed and fasted states. The World Health Organization has set clear guidelines for the condition of diabetes mellitus by defining diabetic hyperglycaemia as fasting and fed blood glucose concentrations rising to, ≥6.1 mmol/l (112 mg/dl) and ≥ 8.1 mmol/l (147 mg/dl) respectively. In contrast, divergent diagnostic criteria have been used to define hyperglycaemia in critically ill patients, resulting in a large variation in the reported prevalence of hyperglycaemia in this group of patients ranging from 3% to 71%.[19] Until recently, it was considered acceptable to tolerate blood glucose levels up to 12 mmol/l (220 mg/dl) in fed critically ill patients.[20] The primary motivation for only treating hyperglycaemia when glucose concentrations exceeded this value was the occurrence of hyperglycaemia-induced osmotic diuresis. Also, fluid shifts once glycaemia crosses this threshold. Secondly, the literature on diabetes demonstrated that uncontrolled and pronounced hyperglycaemia predisposed to infectious complications.[21,22] Another argument for tolerating glucose concentrations up to 12 mmol/l (220 mg/dl) was the common acceptance that moderate hyperglycaemia in critically ill patients is 'beneficial' for organs that largely rely on glucose for their energy supply but do not require insulin for glucose uptake, such as the brain and the blood cells. Finally, moderate hyperglycaemia was viewed as a buffer against the occurrence of hypoglycaemia and brain damage, which was feared by many clinicians to have the potential to occur when a tight glucose control regimen was used.

Strict Maintenance of Normoglycaemia Improves Outcome in Critically Ill Patients

A recent, extensive, prospective, randomized, controlled clinical trial has studied the effects of strict glycaemic control on mortality and morbidity of critically ill patients.[1] The result challenged the classic dogma that stress-induced hyperglycaemia is beneficial to these patients. Over a 1-year period, a total of 1548 patients, admitted to the intensive care unit (ICU) predominantly after extensive or complicated surgery or trauma and requiring mechanical ventilation, were enrolled in the study. The patients were randomly subdivided into two groups. One group received 'intensive insulin therapy' to keep blood glucose concentrations tightly between 4.5 and 6.1 mmol/l (80–110 mg/dl) by exogenous insulin infusion. In contrast, insulin was only administered to the patients in the 'conventional treatment' group if blood glucose levels exceeded 12 mmol/l (220 mg/dl). When normoglycaemia was strictly maintained by intensive insulin therapy, a marked reduction in mortality was observed (Fig. 10.1). The effect was particularly present in the prolonged critically ill patient group with a mortality reduction from 20.2% to 10.6% ($P = 0.005$). The fact that even for patients in the conventional treatment group who showed only moderate hyperglycaemia (6.1–8.3 mmol/l or 110–150 mg/dl) the mortality rate was higher than for intensively treated patients with blood glucose concentrations

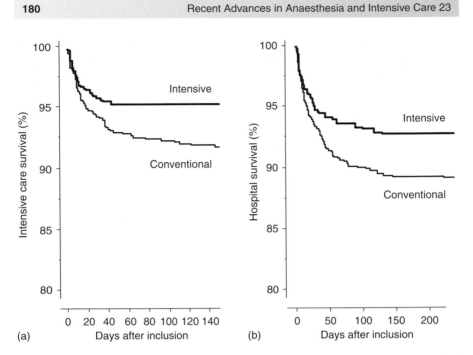

Figure 10.1 Kaplan–Meier cumulative survival plots for intensive care and in-hospital survival showing the effect of intensive insulin treatment in a study of 1548 critically ill patients. Patients discharged alive from intensive care (a) and hospital (b), respectively, were considered survivors. *P*-values were obtained by logrank (Mantel–Cox) significance testing. The difference between the intensive insulin group and the conventional group was significant for intensive care survival (unadjusted $P = 0.005$; adjusted $P < 0.04$) and for hospital survival (unadjusted $P = 0.01$). Reproduced, with permission, from Ref. [1].

<6.1 mmol/l (110 mg/dl), also illustrates the superiority of intensive insulin therapy.[23] The importance of this observation is stressed by the lack of any intervention with such a pronounced beneficial effect on intensive care mortality, since the introduction of mechanical ventilation. Intensive insulin therapy also improved several morbidity-related factors. Thus, the need for prolonged ventilatory support, the duration of intensive care stay, the number of blood transfusions and the incidence of blood stream infections and excessive inflammation were all reduced. Even more striking was the highly significant decrease in the development of acute renal failure and critical illness polyneuropathy associated with intensive insulin therapy.

Complications of Deranged Glucose Regulation

Diabetic patients have improved outcomes with tight glycaemic control

The question whether tight glycaemic control is beneficial for subjects with Type 1 diabetes was the subject of vigorous debate until this issue was resolved in 1993 by the results of the Diabetes Control and Complications

Trial (DCCT). The study demonstrated that maintenance of blood glucose concentrations close to the normal range resulted in a highly significant decrease in the progression rates of not only diabetic retinopathy, the most prevalent complication in Type 1 diabetes, but also in the development of nephropathy, and peripheral and autonomic neuropathy.[24] A large clinical trial provided evidence for the importance of tight glycaemic control in patients with Type 2 diabetes compared with Type 1 diabetes. In the late 1990s, the United Kingdom Prospective Diabetes Study (UKPDS) indeed showed that a 0.7% decrease in glycosylated haemoglobin (HbA1c) following intensive blood glucose control lowered the incidence of retinopathy by 21%, microalbuminuria by 33%, cataract by 24%, myocardial infarction by 16% and resulted in a non-significant 5% decrease in the incidence of cerebrovascular accident.[25] In addition, a tendency towards a lower mortality rate was observed when blood glucose concentrations were tightly controlled. However, neither the UKPDS nor the DCCT were appropriately powered to detect a significant decrease in diabetes-related mortality.

A history of diabetes strongly increases the risk of a fatal outcome following acute myocardial infarction (AMI) with a factor 1.5–2 in comparison to non-diabetic patients.[26] Moreover, in AMI patients without previously diagnosed diabetes, hyperglycaemia on admission has been associated with larger infarction size, a higher incidence of cardiac failure and decreased 1-year survival.[27] The outcome benefits of tightening glycaemic control in diabetic patients with myocardial infarction have been examined by several studies, of which the Diabetes and Insulin–Glucose infusion in Acute Myocardial Infarction (DIGAMI) Study was the largest and also covered the longest follow-up period.[28] In that study, diabetic patients admitted to hospital with an AMI were randomly assigned to standard treatment (at the physician's discretion) or to 'intensive insulin therapy'. An infusion of glucose and insulin was administered to the latter group of patients as soon as possible, and continued for 48 h. Thereafter, the intensive insulin therapy patients were submitted to a 'stricter' blood glucose control regimen (<12 mmol/l or 220 mg/dl) with subcutaneous insulin continued for at least 3 months after discharge. The intensive treatment with insulin significantly improved 30-day and long-term survival (29% relative risk reduction at 1 year)[29,30] and the risk for re-infarction and new cardiac failure was reduced.[31]

Furthermore, for other clinical conditions it has been demonstrated that there is a significant correlation between 'on-admission' hyperglycaemia and adverse outcome. For instance, high blood glucose levels were associated with increased mortality and poorer neurological recovery after cerebrovascular ischaemic insults[32] and mortality of patients with traumatic head injuries appeared to be independently predicted by post-operative hyper-glycaemia.[33] The treatment of patients with glucose–insulin–potassium (GIK) infusion for 24 h after acute stroke was not able to reduce glycaemia or mortality significantly, as examined in the Glucose–Insulin in Stroke Trial (GIST).[34] However, it should be noted that studies on the benefits of GIK infusions in either cardiac or neurological ischaemic insults never targeted normoglycaemia, unlike the insulin schedule in the Leuven ICU Trial. As such they could not provide conclusive evidence as to whether the degree of hyperglycaemia simply reflects the severity of illness or is actually contributing to the adverse outcome of those insults.

Role of hyperglycaemia in critical illness associated renal failure

Presumably, a different pathophysiology is involved in diabetic and critical illness associated nephropathy. In diabetic nephropathy the glomerulus is mainly affected, whereas acute tubular necrosis is the major trigger for renal failure in the critically ill. The prevention of renal function deterioration is of crucial importance to the critically ill patients. The only options for this complication remain prevention or, when this fails, bridging time to spon-taneous recovery by extracorporeal haemofiltration or dialysis, with the continuous veno-venous mode being the preferred method for unstable critic-ally ill patients.[35] Preventive strategies include maintaining or optimizing renal perfusion, diligence with monitoring of nephrotoxic therapies such as aminoglycosides and limiting the use of non-ionic radiocontrast materials. Strikingly, the number of critically ill patients that required extracorporeal replacement therapy to compensate for loss of renal function were reduced by 42% when they were intensively treated with insulin, as compared to the conventionally treated patients. Hence, intensive insulin therapy emerged as an effective preventive measure for acute renal failure in critical illness.

Role of hyperglycaemia in critical illness associated neuropathy

The most frequent presentation of neuropathies in the diabetic patient is dis-tal sensory neuropathy with the classic 'glove-and-stocking' distribution.[36] Protracted critically ill patients often suffer from a diffuse axonal polyneu-ropathy,[37] which presents as a tetraparesis with muscle atrophy, but requires confirmation by electromyography (EMG). Even though the course of crit-ical illness neuropathy is self-limited in most cases and a good recovery should be expected once the underlying critical illness is overcome, it severely delays weaning from the ventilator and impairs early mobilization of the patient.[38] Sepsis, the use of high-dose corticosteroids as well as the use of neuromuscu-lar blocking agents are all factors that have been implicated in the aetiology of critical illness polyneuropathy. Yet, the exact pathogenesis of this complication is still not understood,[39] and this lack of knowledge hampers its specific prevention or treatment. Recently, some indications have emphasized the importance of blood glucose concentrations in relation to the development of critical illness polyneuropathy. Bolton described a strong link between the risk of critical illness polyneuropathy on the one hand, and increased blood glucose and decreased serum albumin concentrations, which are both metabolic manifestations of multiple organ failure and sepsis, on the other. Sepsis, and the accompanying release of cytokines, was considered to be the causal factor.[40] Cytokines may indeed induce microangiopathy, which may play a role as in diabetic polyneuropathy. In addition, the Leuven study on intensive insulin therapy in the ICU convincingly demonstrated that strict maintenance of glycaemia within the normal range by infusion of insulin has an important preventative effect on the incidence of critical illness polyneuropathy, which is associated with a decrease in duration of mechanical ventilation of protracted critically ill patients.[1]

Immune system impairment and risk of infections caused by hyperglycaemia

It is well known that hyperglycaemia of diabetes renders the patient more susceptible to infection.[21] Several mechanisms could account for this phenomenon, including the impairment of interleukin-1 release and phagocytosis by macrophages, and the inhibition of the release of oxygen radicals by neutrophils under hyperglycaemic conditions.[41–43] Importantly, strict glucose control was able to ameliorate the leukocyte oxidative burst and phagocytotic activity.[44,45] In diabetic critically ill patients, such as those after open-heart surgery, an association between higher risk of infectious complications and blood glucose concentrations >11 mmol/l (200 mg/dl) has been documented.[46] A follow-up study demonstrated that the incidence of post-cardiac surgery of deep sternal wounds was reduced by continuous intravenous insulin infusion (0.8% versus 2% for subcutaneous insulin injections).[47] Also, in patients with severe burn injuries, failure of skin graft and outcome seemed to be related to uncontrolled hyperglycaemia.[48] Once more, it was the recent Leuven insulin in ICU study that provided the causal link between hyperglycaemia and higher risk of serious infections, regardless of a previous history of diabetes.[1] Indeed, the occurrence of blood stream infections was reduced by almost 50% and sepsis associated mortality was largely prevented when critically ill patients were intensively treated with exogenous insulin to keep glucose levels within the normal range. Hence, these observations suggest that insulin-titrated blood glucose control enhances the immune system. Improved capacity to clear bacterial invaders was recently shown to mediate this benefit in a novel rabbit model of prolonged critical illness.[49,50]

Impairment of lipid metabolism by critical illness and hyperglycaemia

Deranged metabolism, manifest by hyperglycaemia and by an abnormal lipid profile in serum is observed in both diabetic patients and in critical illness.[51–54] Characteristically, triglyceride levels are elevated, due to an increase in very-low-density lipoprotein (VLDL), and the levels of circulating high-density lipoprotein (HDL) cholesterol are low.[55] The levels of low-density lipoprotein (LDL) cholesterol are also decreased,[55] but this is offset by an increase in circulating small dense LDL particles[56] that presumably are more pro-atherogenic than the medium and large LDL particles.[57] Interestingly, the deranged serum lipid profile during critical illness could partially be restored by intensive insulin therapy, with almost complete obliteration of the hypertriglyceridaemia and a substantial increase in, but not normalisation of, the serum levels of HDL and LDL.[58] The role of triglycerides in energy provision and the co-ordinating position of the lipoproteins in transportation of lipid components (cholesterol, triglycerides, phospholipids and lipid-soluble vitamins) is well established.[59] In addition, it recently has been shown that lipoproteins can scavenge endotoxins and in that way are able to prevent death in animal models.[60,61] For that reason, intensive insulin therapy may improve the overall endotoxin scavenging function. Considering these data, intensive insulin therapy should provide a more integrated approach to correct the abnormal serum lipid profile, in contrast to the proposed infusions of lipoproteins.[55,62] Indeed, multivariate logistic regression analysis demonstrated that the improvement of the deranged lipidaemia explained a significant part of its beneficial effect on mortality and organ failure and, surprisingly, surpassed the effect of glycaemic control and insulin dose. In the same way, the effect of intensive insulin therapy on inflammation, reflected by a lowering of the serum C-reactive protein (CRP) concentrations,[63] was no longer independently related to the outcome benefit when the changes in lipid metabolism were taken into account (see also chapter 8). This observation is suggestive of a link between the anti-inflammatory effect of intensive insulin therapy and its amelioration of the lipid profile. However, a mechanistic explanation for the dominant effect of serum lipid correction still needs to be delineated.

Effects of critical illness and insulin on inflammation and coagulation

Critical illness also resembles diabetes mellitus in the activation of the inflammatory cascade.[64] As for other complications, intensive insulin therapy has proven to be of high value in the prevention of excessive inflammation in critically ill patients subjected to this treatment.[63, 64] This finding was also confirmed in an experimental rabbit model of prolonged critical illness.[50] The exact mechanisms explaining the anti-inflammatory effect of insulin have not yet been unravelled, but several factors may be considered, including suppression of the secretion of tumour necrosis factor-α,[65,66] macrophage migration-inhibitory factor[67] and superoxide, [68] and antagonism of their harmful actions. Furthermore, diabetes mellitus and critical illness both are hypercoagulable states.[69,70] Putative causes in diabetes include vascular endothelium dysfunction,[71] increased blood levels of several clotting factors,[72,73] elevated platelet activation[74,75] and inhibition of the fibrinolytic system.[73] Concentrations of the anticoagulant protein C are also decreased.[76] Looking at the similarities between critical illness and diabetes,[77,78] and the powerful preventive effect of intensive insulin therapy on septicaemia, multiple organ failure and mortality,[1] it is also very important to investigate the influence of this simple and cheap metabolic intervention on the balance between coagulation and fibrinolysis in the critically ill.

Hyper-, normo- or hypocaloric nutrition?
When hypercaloric nutrition (35–40 kcal/kg) is administered to critically ill patients, this condition of 'hyperalimentation' increases the incidence of infections and severe metabolic complications, ranging from hyperglycaemia, hypertriglyceridaemia and azotaemia to hepatic steatosis, fat-overload syndrome and hypertonic dehydration.[79,80] Serious complications of feeding have been reduced due to the availability of more accurate means of estimating energy expenditure. Caution should be used when calculating caloric requirements, particularly in obese or highly oedematous patients.

Comparison of the occurrence of hyperglycaemia and infections under hypocaloric total parenteral nutrition (TPN) feeding (14 kcal/kg) or a standard weight-based regimen (18 kcal/kg) revealed that hypocaloric nutrition did not lower these parameters, as had been expected.[81] Caloric restriction only seems to be effective in conjunction with a hyperproteinic approach (about 1.8 g protein/kg ideal body weight (IBW), compared to 1.2 g/kg IBW).[82] A hypocaloric parenteral regimen with 2 g protein/kg IBW in patients with morbid obesity yielded similar results.[83] However, a clear-cut benefit of hypocaloric over normocaloric nutrition was not consistently present. This might be attributed to the ineffectiveness of hypocaloric nutrition to effectively lower blood glucose levels.

The strategy of combining hypercaloric feeding and insulin infusions, with the aim of enhancing the anabolic effects of insulin, has not been thoroughly investigated, but seems to be promising. Indeed, a meta-analysis of published trials that investigated the effect of GIK infusion in previously non-diabetic subjects with AMI supports the concept that this approach may be of benefit.[84] However, the main goal of GIK infusion is to stimulate myocardial metabolization of glucose instead of fatty acids when oxygen supply is compromised. Interest in pre-operative carbohydrate loading has been rekindled through a recent study by Ljungqvist and colleagues, which revealed that carbohydrate treatment instead of overnight fasting before surgery reduced post-operative insulin resistance and length of hospital stay.[85]

Does a History of Diabetes Imply a Specific Metabolic Management During Critical Illness?

Since the beneficial effect of intensive insulin therapy on morbidity and mortality of critically ill patients was equally present among those with and without previously diagnosed diabetes,[1] the authors believe that strict normoglycaemia <6.1 mmol/l (110 mg/dl) should be the therapeutic goal, regardless of diabetic history. Strict blood glucose control during intensive care can best be attained by continuous insulin infusion for both diabetic and non-diabetic critically ill patients and the use of oral antidiabetic agents should be discontinued during critical illness.

Critically ill patients should be continuously fed by enteral, total parenteral or by a combination of parenteral and enteral nutrition. Therefore, it is logical that insulin should be administered continuously as well. Intravenous administration is preferred to subcutaneous injections because it is more reliable and consistent. In addition, titrating a continuous insulin infusion not only provides a baseline insulin level, but also can be more easily and precisely adjusted in response to the actual blood glucose concentrations. In addition, because of its short intravenous half-life, insulin administration by infusion also allows rapid cessation of insulin action when the patient develops hypoglycaemia.

This risk of hypoglycaemia is a major concern with intensive insulin therapy during critical illness, more so as clinical symptoms of the autonomic response (sweating, tachycardia and tremor) and central nervous symptoms (like dizziness, blurred vision, altered mental acuity, confusion and eventually convulsions) may be masked by concomitant diseases and by inherent intensive care treatments, such as sedation, analgesia and mechanical ventilation. The brain can be irreversibly damaged by severe hypoglycaemia, when blood glucose concentrations decrease to <1.67 mmol/l (30 mg/dl), or in the case of persistent hypoglycaemia. Another insidious complication of hypoglycaemia is the induction of cardiac arrhythmias ranging from increased QT dispersion[86] and sinus bradycardia[87] to ventricular tachycardia.[88]

The administration of insulin together with carbohydrates, either intra-venous dextrose or enteral feeding, as well as close monitoring of blood glucose concentrations are important measures taken to prevent hypogly-caemia in the critically ill. Specifically in the Leuven insulin in ICU study[1] blood glucose concentrations were checked every 1–2 h during the first 12–24 h after the patient's admission to the ICU. Once the targeted blood glucose concentration was reached on a stable insulin dose, measurements were scaled down to every 4 h. When hypoglycaemia developed, it usually took place after the first week of ICU stay at a time when blood glucose concentrations were stable, and was often due to inadequate insulin dose reduction during interruption of enteral feeding. Clearly, the hazard of hypoglycaemia warrants a strict and detailed insulin titration protocol, combined with sufficient training of the nursing and medical staff.

Focus on Insulin or Glycaemic Control?

Data are available in support of the notion that both maintenance of nor-moglycaemia and a direct effect of insulin contribute to the beneficial effects of intensive insulin therapy during critical illness.[1,23] Future studies will help to clarify the exact degree of benefit provided by each.

It is conceivable that insulin plays a direct role in the functional improvement of the insulin-sensitive organs, since in normal individuals the heart and skeletal muscles are responsible for the majority of the insulin-stimulated glucose uptake. Hyperglycaemic conditions aggravate muscle catabolism, thus amelioration of these processes could partially explain the beneficial effects of intensive insulin therapy on duration of mechanical ventilation of critically ill patients. In comparison to the conventional treatment group, skeletal muscle steady-state mRNA concentrations of GLUT-4 and hexokinase II (HXK-II) are higher in patients following intensive insulin therapy. This suggests that peripheral glucose uptake is stimulated in the latter group of patients.[58]

The liver is the major site for gluconeogenesis and also is an important insulin-sensitive organ that could be involved in the improved outcome of patients intensively treated with insulin. However, the analysis of serum and gene expression levels of insulin-like growth factor binding protein-1 (IGFBP-1) and gene expression levels of phosphoenolpyruvate carboxy-kinase (PEPCK), the rate-limiting enzyme in gluconeogenesis, revealed that neither of them is regulated by insulin in critically ill patients. This may indicate that controlling gluconeogenesis is not the major factor responsi-ble for the normalization of blood glucose concentrations with exogenous insulin in the critically ill.[89] However, true glucose kinetics can only be estimated by glucose turnover studies. Nevertheless, such a study, using a well-designed canine model of critical illness, recently endorsed our findings.[90] When a sublethal hypermetabolic infection was induced in the dogs, hepatic glucose uptake was decreased and appeared to be unresponsive to insulin administration. In contrast, the peripheral uptake of glucose did respond to insulin infusion. Contrary to our findings, insulin therapy suppressed hepatic glucose production. This apparently occurred by inhibition of glycogenolysis rather than diminished hepatic uptake of gluconeogenic amino acids and gluconeogenesis.

Another major insulin-responsive organ is adipose tissue. The increased serum free fatty acid and triglyceride concentrations present during critical illness and the relative accretion of adipose tissue as compared with lean body mass (muscle and bone tissue) with feeding in the protracted critically ill patient, jointly point to a deranged lipid metabolism. Intensive insulin therapy was able to partially restore this imbalance in serum lipids, which in turn significantly contributed to the reduced ICU mortality. However, its direct effects on the adipocytes remain to be investigated.[58]

On the other hand, a recent publication by Finney and colleagues showed a positive association between increased insulin administration and death in the ICU, regardless of the prevailing blood glucose concentration.[91] Although this was an observational study mainly confirming the association of insulin resistance and risk of death, the data are in agreement with the previous interpretation[23] that metabolic control, rather than the absolute amount of exogenous insulin, explains the beneficial effect of intensive insulin therapy on mortality.[1]

The positive results regarding renal function and incidence of critical illness polyneuropathy in patients receiving intensive insulin therapy may in part be explained by maintenance of normoglycaemia, as both organs are supposedly, at least in part, insulin insensitive. Again, although on a totally different time scale, a parallel with Type 2 diabetes emerges. Long-term studies have demonstrated that meticulous blood glucose control reduces the incidence and the severity of diabetic nephropathy and the onset of diabetic neuropathy and that 'glucose toxicity' may be the underlying mechanism. Nevertheless, other factors are probably involved, which predispose the critically ill to the toxic effects of hyperglycaemia on neurones and the kidney, since critical illness polyneuropathy and acute renal failure both appear so rapidly. Similarly, avoiding hyperglycaemia may be important for prevention of bloodstream infections. The suppression of the immune system conceivably results in increased risk of post-operative infections, as discussed above. However, the exact underlying mechanisms of the clinical benefits of intensive insulin therapy in critically ill patients remain at this stage unknown. Future clinical and experimental studies will undoubtedly provide the answer to this fascinating pathophysiological question.

Summary

Trauma, burns and critical illness are accompanied by the development of hyperglycaemia, which results from the combined action of hormonal, cytokine and nervous 'counter-regulatory' signals on glucose metabolic pathways. Additionally, the major insulin-sensitive organs become resistant to insulin during critical illness, as manifested by increased serum insulin levels, impaired peripheral glucose uptake and elevated hepatic glucose production.[18] Recently, Van den Berghe and colleagues demonstrated the beneficial effects of strictly maintaining normoglycaemia in ICU patients by administration of intensive insulin therapy.[1] A significant reduction in mortality of ICU patients was observed, particularly of those with prolonged critical illness. Furthermore, intensive insulin therapy was able to protect against acute renal failure and the development of critical illness polyneuropathy; and also partially counteracted the deranged serum lipid profile, excessive inflammation and impaired immunity seen in critically ill patients.

The authors believe that blood glucose levels in critically ill patients should be tightly controlled between 4.5 and 6.1 mmol/l (80–110 mg/dl) by continuous infusion of insulin, irrespective of underlying diabetes. Blood sugar concentration should be measured every 1–2 h until stable and then reduced to 4-h intervals. Caution must be taken when infusing intravenous insulin in order to eliminate the possibility of hypoglycaemic complications, particularly whenever feeding is interrupted. In addition, oral antidiabetic agents should be discontinued during critical illness.

References

1. Van den Berghe G, Wouters P, Weekers F et al. Intensive insulin therapy in critically ill patients. New Engl J Med 2001; 345: 1359–1367.
2. Hill M, McCallum R. Altered transcriptional regulation of phosphoenolpyruvate carboxykinase in rats following endotoxin treatment. J Clin Invest 1991; 88: 811–816.
3. Khani S, Tayek JA. Cortisol increases gluconeogenesis in humans: its role in the metabolic syndrome. Clin Sci (Lond) 2001; 101: 739–747.
4. Watt MJ, Howlett KF, Febbraio MA, Spriet LL, Hargreaves M. Adrenaline increases skeletal muscle glycogenolysis, pyruvate dehydrogenase activation and carbohydrate oxidation during moderate exercise in humans. J Physiol 2001; 534: 269–278.

5. Flores EA, Istfan N, Pomposelli JJ, Blackburn GL, Bistrian BR. Effect of interleukin-1 and tumor necrosis factor/cachectin on glucose turnover in the rat. Metabolism 1990; 39: 738–743.

6. Sakurai Y, Zhang XJ, Wolfe RR. TNF directly stimulates glucose uptake and leucine oxidation and inhibits FFA flux in conscious dogs. Am J Physiol 1996; 270: E864–E872.

7. Lang CH, Dobrescu C, Bagby GJ. Tumor necrosis factor impairs insulin action on peripheral glucose disposal and hepatic glucose output. Endocrinology 1992; 130: 43–52.

8. Van den Berghe G, de Zegher F, Bouillon R. Clinical review 95: acute and prolonged critical illness as different neuroendocrine paradigms. J Clin Endocrinol Metab 1998; 83: 1827–1834.

9. Damas P, Reuter A, Gysen P, Demonty J, Lamy M, Franchimon P. Tumor necrosis factor and interleukin-1 serum levels during severe sepsis in humans. Crit Care Med 1989; 17: 975–978.

10. Van den Berghe G, Weekers F, Baxter RC, Wouters P, Iranmanesh A, Bouillon R, Veldhuis JD. Five-day pulsatile gonadotropin-releasing hormone administration unveils combined hypothalamic–pituitary–gonadal defects underlying profound hypoandrogenism in men with prolonged critical illness. J Clin Endocrinol Metab 2001; 86: 3217–3226.

11. Stephens JM, Bagby GJ, Pekala PH, Shepherd RE, Spitzer JJ, Lang CH. Differential regulation of glucose transporter gene expression in adipose tissue or septic rats. Biochem Biophys Res Commun 1992; 183: 417–422.

12. Virkamaki A, Yki-Jarvinen H. Mechanisms of insulin resistance during acute endotoxemia. Endocrinology 1994; 134: 2072–2078.

13. Stoner HB, Little RA, Frayn KN, Elebute AE, Tresadern J, Gross E. The effect of sepsis on the oxidation of carbohydrate and fat. Br J Surg 1983; 70: 32–35.

14. Gore DC, Jahoor F, Hibbert JM, DeMaria EJ. Lactic acidosis during sepsis is related to increased pyruvate production, not deficits in tissue oxygen availability. Ann Surg 1996; 224: 97–102.

15. Meszaros K, Lang CH, Bagby GJ, Spitzer JJ. In vivo glucose utilization by individual tissues during nonlethal hypermetabolic sepsis. FASEB J 1988; 2: 3083–3086.

16. Meszaros K, Lang CH, Bagby GJ, Spitzer JJ. Contribution of different organs to increased glucose consumption after endotoxin administration. J Biol Chem 1987; 262: 10965–10970.

17. Long CL, Schiller WR, Geiger JW, Blakemore WS. Gluconeogenic response during glucose infusions in patients following skeletal trauma or during sepsis. J Parenter Enteral Nutr 1978; 2: 619–626.

18. Mizock BA. Alterations in fuel metabolism in critical illness: hyperglycaemia. Best Pract Res Clin Endocrinol Metab 2001; 15: 533–551.

19. Capes SE, Hunt D, Malmberg K, Gerstein HC. Stress hyperglycaemia and increased risk of death after myocardial infarction in patients with and without diabetes: a systematic overview. Lancet 2000; 355: 773–778.

20. Boord JB, Graber AL, Christman JW, Powers AC. Practical management of diabetes in critically ill patients. Am J Respir Crit Care Med 2001; 164: 1763–1767.

21. Pozzilli P, Leslie RD. Infections and diabetes: mechanisms and prospects for prevention. Diabet Med 1994; 11: 935–941.

22. McCowen KC, Malhotra A, Bistrian BR. Stress-induced hyperglycaemia. Crit Care Clin 2001; 17: 107–124.

23. Van den Berghe G, Wouters PJ, Bouillon R *et al*. Outcome benefit of intensive insulin therapy in the critically ill: insulin dose versus glycemic control. Crit Care Med 2003; 31: 359–366.
24. The Diabetes Control and Complications Trial Research Group. The effect of intensive treatment of diabetes on the development and progression of long-term complications in insulin-dependent diabetes mellitus. New Engl J Med 1993; 329: 977–986.
25. UK Prospective Diabetes Study (UKPDS) Group. Intensive blood-glucose control with sulphonylureas or insulin compared with conventional treatment and risk of complications in patients with type 2 diabetes (UKPDS 33). Lancet 1998; 352: 837–853.
26. Mukamal KJ, Nesto RW, Cohen MC, Muller JE, Maclure M, Sherwood JB, Mittleman MA. Impact of diabetes on long-term survival after acute myocardial infarction: comparability of risk with prior myocardial infarction. Diabetes Care 2001; 24: 1422–1427.
27. Bolk J, van der Ploeg T, Cornel JH, Arnold AE, Sepers J, Umans VA. Impaired glucose metabolism predicts mortality after a myocardial infarction. Int J Cardiol 2001; 79: 207–214.
28. Malmberg K, McGuire DK. Diabetes and acute myocardial infarction: the role of insulin therapy. Am Heart J 1999; 138: S381–S386.
29. Malmberg K, Ryden L, Efendic S *et al*. Randomized trial of insulin-glucose infusion followed by subcutaneous insulin treatment in diabetic patients with acute myocardial infarction (DIGAMI study): effects on mortality at 1 year. J Am Coll Cardiol 1995; 26: 57–65.
30. Malmberg K. Prospective randomised study of intensive insulin treatment on long-term survival after acute myocardial infarction in patients with diabetes mellitus. DIGAMI (Diabetes Mellitus, Insulin Glucose Infusion in Acute Myocardial Infarction) Study Group. Br Med J 1997; 314: 1512–1515.
31. Malmberg K, Ryden L, Hamsten A, Herlitz J, Waldenstrom A, Wedel H. Effects of insulin treatment on cause-specific one-year mortality and morbidity in diabetic patients with acute myocardial infarction. DIGAMI Study Group. Diabetes Insulin–Glucose in Acute Myocardial Infarction. Eur Heart J 1996; 17: 1337–1344.
32. Williams LS, Rotich J, Qi R *et al*. Effects of admission hyperglycaemia on mortality and costs in acute ischemic stroke. Neurology 2002; 59: 67–71.
33. Rovlias A, Kotsou S. The influence of hyperglycaemia on neurological outcome in patients with severe head injury. Neurosurgery 2000; 46: 335–342; discussion 342–343.
34. Scott JF, Robinson GM, French JM, O'Connell JE, Alberti KG, Gray CS. Glucose potassium insulin infusions in the treatment of acute stroke patients with mild to moderate hyperglycaemia: the Glucose Insulin in Stroke Trial (GIST). Stroke 1999; 30: 793–799.
35. Murray P, Hall J. Renal replacement therapy for acute renal failure. Am J Respir Crit Care Med 2000; 162: 777–781.
36. Boulton AJ. Clinical presentation and management of diabetic neuropathy and foot ulceration. Diabet Med 1991; 8: S52–S57.
37. Hund E. Neurological complications of sepsis: critical illness polyneuropathy and myopathy. J Neurol 2001; 248: 929–934.
38. Leijten FS, De Weerd AW, Poortvliet DC, De Ridder VA, Ulrich C, Harink-De Weerd JE. Critical illness polyneuropathy in multiple organ dysfunction

syndrome and weaning from the ventilator. Intens Care Med 1996; 22: 856–861.

39. Bolton CF, Young GB. Critical illness polyneuropathy. Curr Treat Option Neurol 2000; 2: 489–498.

40. Bolton CF. Sepsis and the systemic inflammatory response syndrome: neuro-muscular manifestations. Crit Care Med 1996; 24: 1408–1416.

41. Nielson CP, Hindson DA. Inhibition of polymorphonuclear leukocyte respiratory burst by elevated glucose concentrations in vitro. Diabetes 1989; 38: 1031–1035.

42. Kwoun MO, Ling PR, Lydon E, Imrich A, Qu Z, Palombo J, Bistrian BR. Immunologic effects of acute hyperglycaemia in nondiabetic rats. J Parenter Enteral Nutr 1997; 21: 91–95.

43. Rassias AJ, Marrin CA, Arruda J, Whalen PK, Beach M, Yeager MP. Insulin infusion improves neutrophil function in diabetic cardiac surgery patients. Anesth Analg 1999; 88: 1011–1016.

44. Rayfield EJ, Ault MJ, Keusch GT, Brothers MJ, Nechemias C, Smith H. Infection and diabetes: the case for glucose control. Am J Med 1982; 72: 439–450.

45. Rassias AJ, Givan AL, Marrin CA, Whalen PK, Pahl J, Yeager MP. Insulin increases neutrophil count and phagocytic capacity after cardiac surgery. Anesth Analg 2002; 94: 1113–1119.

46. Zerr KJ, Furnary AP, Grunkemeier GL, Bookin S, Kanhere V, Starr A. Glucose control lowers the risk of wound infection in diabetics after open heart operations. Ann Thorac Surg 1997; 63: 356–361.

47. Furnary AP, Zerr KJ, Grunkemeier GL, Starr A. Continuous intravenous insulin infusion reduces the incidence of deep sternal wound infection in diabetic patients after cardiac surgical procedures. Ann Thorac Surg 1999; 67: 352–360; discussion 360–362.

48. Gore DC, Chinkes D, Heggers J, Herndon DN, Wolf SE, Desai M. Association of hyperglycaemia with increased mortality after severe burn injury. J Trauma 2001; 51: 540–544.

49. Weekers F, Van Herck E, Coopmans W, Michalaki M, Bowers CY, Veldhuis JD, Van den Berghe G. A novel in vivo rabbit model of hypercatabolic critical illness reveals a biphasic neuroendocrine stress response. Endocrinology 2002; 143: 764–774.

50. Weekers F, Giulietti A, Michalaki M, Coopmans W, Van Herck E, Mathieu C, Van den Berghe G. Metabolic, endocrine and immune effects of stress hyperglycaemia in a rabbit model of prolonged critical illness. Endocrinology 2003; 144: 5329–5338.

51. Taskinen MR. Pathogenesis of dyslipidemia in type 2 diabetes. Exp Clin Endocrinol Diabetes 2001; 109: S180–S188.

52. Lanza-Jacoby S, Wong SH, Tabares A, Baer D, Schneider T. Disturbances in the composition of plasma lipoproteins during gram-negative sepsis in the rat. Biochim Biophys Acta 1992; 1124: 233–240.

53. Khovidhunkit W, Memon RA, Feingold KR, Grunfeld C. Infection and inflammation-induced proatherogenic changes of lipoproteins. J Infect Dis 2000; 181: S462–S472.

54. Carpentier YA, Scruel O. Changes in the concentration and composition of plasma lipoproteins during the acute phase response. Curr Opin Clin Nutr Metab Care 2002; 5: 153–158.

55. Gordon BR, Parker TS, Levine DM et al. Low lipid concentrations in critical illness: implications for preventing and treating endotoxemia. Crit Care Med 1996; 24: 584–589.

56. Feingold KR, Krauss RM, Pang M, Doerrler W, Jensen P, Grunfeld C. The hypertriglyceridemia of acquired immunodeficiency syndrome is associated with an increased prevalence of low density lipoprotein subclass pattern B. J Clin Endocrinol Metab 1993; 76: 1423–1427.
57. Kwiterovich Jr PO. Lipoprotein heterogeneity: diagnostic and therapeutic implications. Am J Cardiol 2002; 90: 1i–10i.
58. Mesotten D, Swinnen JV, Vanderhoydonc F, Wouters PJ, Van den Berghe G. The relative contribution of lipid and glucose control to the improved outcome of critical illness obtained by intensive insulin therapy. J Clin Endocrinol Metab 2004; 89: 219–226.
59. Tulenko TN, Sumner AE. The physiology of lipoproteins. J Nucl Cardiol 2002; 9: 638–649.
60. Harris HW, Grunfeld C, Feingold KR, Rapp JH. Human very low density lipoproteins and chylomicrons can protect against endotoxin-induced death in mice. J Clin Invest 1990; 86: 696–702.
61. Harris HW, Grunfeld C, Feingold KR et al. Chylomicrons alter the fate of endotoxin, decreasing tumor necrosis factor release and preventing death. J Clin Invest 1993; 91: 1028–1034.
62. Harris HW, Johnson JA, Wigmore SJ. Endogenous lipoproteins impact the response to endotoxin in humans. Crit Care Med 2002; 30: 23–31.
63. Hansen TK, Thiel S, Wouters PJ, Christiansen JS, Van den Berghe G. Intensive insulin therapy exerts antiinflammatory effects in critically ill patients and counteracts the adverse effect of low mannose-binding lectin levels. J Clin Endocrinol Metab 2003; 88: 1082–1088.
64. Das UN. Is insulin an antiinflammatory molecule? Nutrition 2001; 17: 409–413.
65. Satomi N, Sakurai A, Haranaka K. Relationship of hypoglycaemia to tumor necrosis factor production and antitumor activity: role of glucose, insulin, and macrophages. J Natl Cancer Inst 1985; 74: 1255–1260.
66. Fraker DL, Merino MJ, Norton JA. Reversal of the toxic effects of cachectin by concurrent insulin administration. Am J Physiol 1989; 256: E725–E731.
67. Sakaue S, Nishihira J, Hirokawa J et al. Regulation of macrophage migration inhibitory factor (MIF) expression by glucose and insulin in adipocytes in vitro. Mol Med 1999; 5: 361–371.
68. Chen HC, Guh JY, Shin SJ, Tsai JH, Lai YH. Insulin and heparin suppress superoxide production in diabetic rat glomeruli stimulated with low-density lipoprotein. Kidney Int Suppl 2001; 78: S124–S127.
69. Carr ME. Diabetes mellitus: a hypercoagulable state. J Diabetes Complications 2001; 15: 44–54.
70. Calles-Escandon J, Garcia-Rubi E, Mirza S, Mortensen A. Type 2 diabetes: one disease, multiple cardiovascular risk factors. Coronary Artery Dis 1999; 10: 23–30.
71. Williams E, Timperley WR, Ward JD, Duckworth T. Electron microscopical studies of vessels in diabetic peripheral neuropathy. J Clin Pathol 1980; 33: 462–470.
72. Patrassi GM, Vettor R, Padovan D, Girolami A. Contact phase of blood coagulation in diabetes mellitus. Eur J Clin Invest 1982; 12: 307–311.
73. Carmassi F, Morale M, Puccetti R, De Negri F, Monzani F, Navalesi R, Mariani G. Coagulation and fibrinolytic system impairment in insulin dependent diabetes mellitus. Thromb Res 1992; 67: 643–654.
74. Hughes A, McVerry BA, Wilkinson L, Goldstone AH, Lewis D, Bloom A. Diabetes, a hypercoagulable state? Hemostatic variables in newly diagnosed type 2 diabetic patients. Acta Haematol 1983; 69: 254–259.

75. Garcia Frade LJ, de la Calle H, Alava I, Navarro JL, Creighton LJ, Gaffney PJ. Diabetes mellitus as a hypercoagulable state: its relationship with fibrin fragments and vascular damage. Thromb Res 1987; 47: 533–540.
76. Vukovich TC, Schernthaner G. Decreased protein C levels in patients with insulin-dependent type I diabetes mellitus. Diabetes 1986; 35: 617–619.
77. Garcia Frade LJ, Landin L, Avello AG, Martin Yerro J, Navarro JL, Creighton LJ, Gaffney PJ. Changes in fibrinolysis in the intensive care patient. Thromb Res 1987; 47: 593–599.
78. Mavrommatis AC, Theodoridis T, Economou M, Kotanidou A, El Ali M, Christopoulou-Kokkinou V, Zakynthinos SG. Activation of the fibrinolytic system and utilization of the coagulation inhibitors in sepsis: comparison with severe sepsis and septic shock. Intens Care Med 2001; 27: 1853–1859.
79. Schloerb PR, Henning JF. Patterns and problems of adult total parenteral nutrition use in US academic medical centers. Arch Surg 1998; 133: 7–12.
80. Klein CJ, Stanek GS, Wiles III CE. Overfeeding macronutrients to critically ill adults: metabolic complications. J Am Diet Assoc 1998; 98: 795–806.
81. McCowen KC, Friel C, Sternberg J, Chan S, Forse RA, Burke PA, Bistrian BR. Hypocalorific total parenteral nutrition: effectiveness in prevention of hyperglycaemia and infectious complications – a randomized clinical trial. Crit Care Med 2000; 28: 3606–3611.
82. Patino JF, de Pimiento SE, Vergara A, Savino P, Rodriguez M, Escallon J. Hypocalorific support in the critically ill. World J Surg 1999; 23: 553–559.
83. Choban PS, Burge JC, Scales D, Flancbaum L. Hypoenergetic nutrition support in hospitalized obese patients: a simplified method for clinical application. Am J Clin Nutr 1997; 66: 546–550.
84. Fath-Ordoubadi F, Beatt KJ. Glucose–insulin–potassium therapy for treatment of acute myocardial infarction: an overview of randomized placebo-controlled trials. Circulation 1997; 96: 1152–1156.
85. Soop M, Nygren J, Myrenfors P, Thorell A, Ljungqvist O. Preoperative oral carbohydrate treatment attenuates immediate postoperative insulin resistance. Am J Physiol Endocrinol Metab 2001; 280: E576–E583.
86. Landstedt-Hallin L, Englund A, Adamson U, Lins PE. Increased QT dispersion during hypoglycaemia in patients with type 2 diabetes mellitus. J Intern Med 1999; 246: 299–307.
87. Pollock G, Brady Jr WJ, Hargarten S, DeSilvey D, Carner CT. Hypoglycaemia manifested by sinus bradycardia: a report of three cases. Acad Emerg Med 1996; 3: 700–707.
88. Chelliah YR. Ventricular arrhythmias associated with hypoglycaemia. Anaesth Intens Care 2000; 28: 698–700.
89. Mesotten D, Delhanty PJD, Vanderhoydonc F, Hardman KV, Weekers F, Baxter RC, Van den Berghe G. Regulation of insulin-like growth factor binding protein-1 during protracted critical illness. J Clin Endocrinol Metab 2002; 87: 5516–5523.
90. Donmoyer CM, Chen SS, Lacy DB, Pearson DA, Poole A, Zhang Y, McGuinnes OP. Infection impairs insulin-dependent hepatic glucose uptake during total parenteral nutrition. Am J Physiol Endocrinol Metab 2003; 284: E574–E582.
91. Finney SJ, Zekveld C, Elia A, Evans TW. Glucose control and mortality in critically ill patients. J Am Med Assoc 2003; 290: 2041–2047.

J. Jage   F. Heid

Substance use disorders and anaesthesia

Anaesthesia and postoperative analgesia in patients dependent on psychoactive substances poses special problems. Often these patients suffer from severe medical and psychiatric illness. In addition drug-specific adaptations such as tolerance, physical dependence and withdrawal may diminish the effectiveness of anaesthetic and analgesic drugs. However, the problem of dependence on psychoactive substances affects health care providers as well as patients. One in 15 doctors in the UK may suffer from some form of dependence on alcohol or drugs during their lifetime[1] and anaesthetists are three times more likely to become substance abusers than other physician groups (www.asahq.org//curricrevFINAL040501.htm). In order to provide adequate care for patients dependent on psychoactive substances the following issues should be taken into consideration:

- Basic aspects of substance use disorders (SUD).

- Clinical aspects of SUD.
  - SUD with central nervous system (CNS)-depressant substances.
  - SUD with CNS-stimulant substances.

- Patients in drug-free recovery.

Basic Aspects of Substance Use Disorders (SUD)

Substance dependence is a maladaptive pattern of substance abuse, leading to clinically significant impairment or distress. According to the *Diagnostic and Statistical Manual of Mental Disorders* (DSM-IV) SUD comprise two

---

Table 11.1 Modified diagnostic criteria of substance dependence

- Tolerance
- Physical dependence
- Substance taken in larger amounts and over a longer period than intended
- Persistent desire to control substance abuse
- A great deal of time is necessary to obtain the substance or recover from its effects
- Important social, occupational or recreational activities are given up/reduced
- Substance abuse despite knowledge of harm

Adapted from Ref. 2.

---

main groups: substance dependence/abuse disorders and substance-induced disorders (viz. intoxication, withdrawal, delirium, psychotic disorders).[2] Three or more diagnostic criteria occurring at any time in the same 12-month period are necessary for a diagnosis of SUD (Table 11.1). SUD is a chronic neurobiological disease and factors influencing drug abuse and dependence include:

- Pharmacological factors.

- Psychosocial factors.

- Genetic factors.

- Environmental factors.

Some useful SUD-related definitions are listed in the Appendix.

Psychoactive substances have a well-defined addiction potential,[3] caused by the predominant dopaminergic rewarding pathway in the mesocorticolimbic system[4,5] with compulsive behaviour as the core symptom of addiction.[6] Natural rewards (food, drink and sex) as well as drugs of addiction stimulate the release of dopamine. Dopamine mediates the hedonistic consequences of a reinforcing stimulus, promoting learning/anticipation of rewarding effects. Addiction can be viewed, therefore, as a form of drug-induced long-term neural and behavioural plasticity.[5] Dopamine receptors, opioid receptors, cannabinoid receptors and serotonin 5-HT$_{2A}$ receptors are all G-protein-coupled (metabotropic) receptors and drug-induced adaptations in the efficacy of receptor/G-protein coupling may contribute to tolerance and sensitization. Furthermore, alcohol and hallucinogens are partial agonists at the serotonin 5-HT$_{2A}$ receptor while cocaine and other stimulants enhance dopamine-mediated neurotransmission by blocking dopamine re-uptake. Cocaine cravings during detoxification are decreased by the dopamimetic agent bromocriptine whereas the dopamine agonist methylphenidate increases rather than decreases cravings. Upregulation of the cAMP second messenger pathway occurs in many neuronal cell types in response to chronic exposure to opioids and other drugs of abuse. Upregulation results in activation of the transcription factor cAMP-responsive element-binding protein (CREB), which mediates tolerance and dependence. Thus, regulation of neural gene expression may be involved in the process by which drugs of abuse cause a state of addiction.[5] Short-term opioid administration activates the G-protein-coupled μ receptor inhibiting adenyl cyclase and thus reducing cAMP, which in turn reduces phosphorylation of CREB and the transcription factor ΔFosB. Whereas continuous stimulation of the opioid receptor results in upregulation of the transcriptional factor β-arrestin which binds to the receptor causing internalization resulting in desensitization of the receptor.[5] Far less is known about inhalant (solvent) abuse. The cellular basis for abuse of the volatile alkyl nitrates probably resides in a direct action on smooth muscle to produce vasodilatation, but a direct effect on the brain cannot be ruled out. There is evidence that the prototypic abused volatile solvent toluene inhibits glutamatergic neurotransmission involving the N-methyl-D-aspartate (NMDA) receptor. However, toluene has also been shown to have some dopaminergic effects.[7]

The interactions between psychoactive substances, psychological influences and social influences may be more important for the development of an active dependence than the exposure to the chemical substance alone.[4] The lifetime prevalence of alcohol dependence in the non-institutionalized civilian population of the US is 20.1% for men and 8.2% for women, [8] while for illicit drug use it is 7.7% for men and 4.8% for women.[9] The 12-month prevalence of any substance abuse/dependence is 16.1% for men and 6.6% for women.[8] Furthermore, the prevalence among patients with SUD of psychiatric illness, such as affective disorders (viz. major depression, phobias, anxiety and somatoform disorders), and personality disorders (viz. borderline or antisocial behaviour), is much higher than in the normal population.[8] Psychiatric illness increases pain intensities and reduces the compliance of patients.[10–12] The number of polydrug abusers with multiple organic diseases is increasing.[4,13,14] In patients with severe SUD a high incidence of infectious diseases such as human immunodeficiency virus (HIV), tuberculosis, hepatitis A, B and C, has been observed, all involving an increased risk of infection for staff members (Table 11.2). The intensity of SUD varies according to the psychotropic substance.[4] CNS-depressant substances such as opioids, alcohol, etc., induce severe

Table 11.2 Preoperative morbidity in patients with SUD

System	Symptom/disease
Cardiovascular system	Cardiomyopathy, valvular diseases, endocarditis, coronary sclerosis, thromboembolic complications **Cocaine:** myocardial ischaemia, infarction, aortic dissection
Blood vessels	Thrombophlebitis, sclerosed vessels, septic embolization, accidental intraarterial injection with severe arterial spastic reaction
Pulmonary system	Chronic obstructive/restrictive disease, pulmonary hypertension, infection **Opioids:** pulmonary embolism **Cocaine:** pneumothorax, pneumomediastinum
Nervous system	Polyneuropathy, encephalopathy, myelitis, parkinsonism **Cocaine:** intracranial haematoma, pontine myolysis
Behavioural/psychiatric disorder	Anxiety, depression, psychosis, disorientation, hallucination, schizophrenia, personality disorders, compulsive behaviour, danger of suicide **Cocaine and amphetamine** (after acute drug action): sleepiness, fatigue **Alcohol:** delirium tremens
Nutrition	Malnutrition
Liver	Hepatitis A, B, C, cirrhosis, coagulopathy **Cocaine:** cholinesterase deficiency
Pancreas	Pancreatitis
Kidney	Nephropathy, pyelonephritis
Skin	Abscess, scars, track marks, burns, phlebitis
Muscles	Myopathy **Opioids, cocaine** (intoxication): danger of rhabdomyolysis
Spine	**Opioids:** osteomyelitis, radicular symptoms
Haematopoetic system	**Alcohol:** anaemia (normochromic, hypochromic, megaloblastic) **Cocaine:** thrombocytopathy
Immune system	Mutiple infections: abscess, endocarditis, pneumonia, tuberculosis, HIV, tetanus, parasites
Sexually transmitted diseases	HIV, syphilis, gonorrhoea, trichomonas

psychological and physical dependence associated with a high degree of tolerance, whereas CNS-stimulant substances, such as cocaine, induce severe psychological dependence with little or no physical dependence or tolerance.[15,16] Patients exhibit compulsive behaviour, craving, chronic psychiatric comorbidity, mental instability, low compliance and different organic illness (Table 11.2). Additional phenomena such as physical dependence and tolerance can influence the perioperative management of these patients.

Definitions

Physical dependence

Physical dependence is not the same as psychological dependence. Physical dependence is only associated with the abuse of CNS-depressant substances such as opioid drugs, alcohol, benzodiazepines and barbiturates, but not with CNS-stimulant substances such as cocaine and amphetamine.[15] Physical withdrawal symptoms occur if the substance is abruptly withdrawn or its dose is too low, but subside after readministration of the substance.[17] The different withdrawal symptoms may be stressful and life-threatening.[18-20] Onset depends on the time of last substance exposure as well as on pharmacokinetic aspects.[15] Administration of the withdrawn substance (substitution) or of a similarly acting substance (cross dependence) terminates withdrawal symptoms quickly.[21] Acute withdrawal of CNS-depressant substances increases perioperative stress and should be avoided during the immediate postoperative period. Predominantly affective withdrawal symptoms associated with craving behaviour are observed after discontinuation of CNS-stimulant substances such as cocaine and amphetamines.[14-16] However, the mild physical withdrawal symptoms are of little clinical significance.[15]

Tolerance

Structural changes of opioid receptors (downregulation, lysosomal degradation and degree of internalisation [see chapter 2]) as well as neuronal adaptations (activation of NMDA and cholecystokinin receptors, increasing activity of adenylcyclases and protein kinases) counteract the primary effects of the substance of abuse causing not only physical dependence, but also tolerance.[5,6,22] The latent hyperexcitability due to neuronal and subcellular counter regulations can turn into hyperalgesia[5,23-25] with increasing intra- and postoperative nociception and, therefore, intensified circulatory, endocrine, gastrointestinal and other responses.

Tolerance and physical dependence can be severe especially in polydrug users, and may result in decreased effectiveness of opioid analgesia.[5] Thus, SUD patients need higher dosages of opioids than non-dependent patients.[19,26,27,27a] On the other hand tolerance to the central effects (viz. sedation and ventilatory depression), ensures safety even with high doses of opioids.[16,26-28] High dose methadone can induce ventricular dysrhythmias.[29] The absence of cross tolerance between alcohol, benzodiazepines, cocaine, amphetamines and cannabis on the one hand and opioid drugs on the other explains why it is possible to apply an analgesic dosage regimen in the same way as in patients without SUD.[15] Psychological factors may increase the demand for opioid analgesic but do not represent tolerance to side effects as with opioid-dependent patients.[30]

Clinical Aspects of SUD

Organ damage is common in dependent patients and extensive preoperative investigation with blood and urine drug screening is necessary to exclude acute drug exposure without clinical symptoms (Table 11.2).[31-33] In addition the higher risk of organic and psychological complications in patients with SUD necessitates intensive postoperative monitoring after major surgery and after severe trauma.[19,31-33]

Well-organized perioperative management is necessary to prevent stressful withdrawal symptoms.[19,34,35] Early interdisciplinary communication is important. Either general anaesthesia without the new opioid remifentanil[75] or regional anaesthesia may be employed (Table 11.3). However, regional anaesthetic techniques are associated with lower pain intensity compared with systemic analgesia.[36] Regional anaesthesia may, therefore, be preferred as it diminishes perioperative stress and improves outcome especially when employed as part of an integrated, multimodal technique with intensive rehabilitation, mobilization and early discharge.[37] Analgesic undertreatment or withdrawal should be avoided (Table 11.4). If possible, the opioid dosage should be gradually reduced before discharge. However, most patients with SUD are non-compliant and tend to leave the hospital as soon as possible.

The perioperative management should focus on three key issues:

- Estimation of organic and psychiatric illness.
- Stabilization of SUD and prevention of withdrawal symptoms.
- Provision of safe and effective anaesthesia and analgesia.

SUD with CNS-depressant Substances

Heroin and other opioids

The degree of psychological and physical dependence is usually severe as is the extent of pre-existing organ damage (Table 11.2).[32] In addition to baseline opioid therapy to prevent withdrawal these patients also need high doses of opioid for analgesia during the perioperative period. Factors influencing the choice of anaesthesia are outlined in Table 11.3.

Pain relief is problematic in opioid-dependent patients but ineffective pain relief may result in severe behavioural disturbances.[12] Factors influencing the choice of analgesic therapy are outlined in Table 11.4. Regional analgesic techniques have advantages over systemic analgesia.[19,27a,36,37] Therapy

Table 11.3 Anaesthesia in patients with SUD

Prophylaxis of physical withdrawal symptoms
- Premedication (benzodiazepines; in patients with SUD with opiods: methadone)

Modifications of anaesthesia technique
Regional anaesthesia
- Regional anaesthesia preferred especially use of catheter techniques but avoid in very anxious/nervous patients or with usual contraindications

General anaesthesia
- Avoid succinylcholine (rhabdomyolysis) and halothane (hepatic damage)
- Isoflurane, desflurane, sevoflurane can all be used
- High doses of opioids (sufentanil, fentanyl) acceptable but avoid remifentanil (induction of postoperative hyperalgesia[73–75] with catastrophic increasing pain and sympathetic stimulation)
- Total intravenous anaesthesia is possible (but with opioids other than remifentanil)
- Avoid antagonists (neostigmine, flumazenil, naloxone)
- Use additional regional anaesthetic techniques (infiltrations, catheters)
- Use intravenous non-opioids shortly before the end of anaesthesia (paracetamol, NSAID)

Table 11.4 Analgesic management of patients with SUD

Systemic analgesia
- Non-opioids: NSAID, acetaminophen, dipyrone; if necessary spasmolytics
  Application: intravenous, rectal, oral
- Opioids (depending on pain intensity)

SUD with heroin or other opioids
- Use only μ-agonist opioids at high doses as short-acting analgesics, for example morphine, piritramide, etc.
- Avoid partial agonists such as buprenorphine, and agonists–antagonists such as pentazocine
- Application: intravenous (PCA with background infusion or continuous infusion), subcutaneous, intramuscular, rectal, oral

SUD with alcohol, benzodiazpine, cocaine, amphetamine, cannabis, LSD
- For mild to moderate pain use tramadol
- For severe pain use morphine, piritramide, etc. Buprenorphine is possible but at higher doses is less effective as an analgesic compared with μ-agonist opioids
- Application: intravenous (PCA without background infusion), subcutaneous, intramuscular, rectal, oral

Regional analgesia
- Use catheter techniques whenever possible (epidural, femoral, brachial plexus, sciatic, others)
- Alternatively intraoperative infiltration/instillation (tissue, nerves)
- *Drugs*: Local anaesthetics (ropivacaine, levo-bupivacaine) plus opioids (morphine, fentanyl, sufentanil: epidural analgesia) plus clonidine (epidural analgesia, peripheral nerve analgesia)
  Application: continuous regional infusion or regional PCA with background infusion
- Adapted administration of NSAID, acetaminophen, dipyrone; if necessary spasmolytics
  Application: intravenous, rectal, oral

with high doses of opioid for example with intravenous patient-controlled analgesia (PCA) does not necessarily imply an aggravation of SUD, rather a transient stabilization of both psychological and physical dependence.[19,26–27] Balanced analgesia with non-opioids (paracetamol [acetaminophen], non-steroidal anti-inflammatory drugs (NSAIDs) and dipyrone) is equally as valuable as in patients without opioid dependence.[26–27] The integration of analgesic therapy and early postoperative mobilization and early ambulation (fast track) is important.[37]

Withdrawal prophylaxis and treatment

As the symptoms of opioid withdrawal vary considerably the opioid withdrawal scale (OWS) was developed in an attempt to quantify the severity of withdrawal.[38] The most effective treatment for opioid dependence is opioid agonist therapy but opioid antagonist therapy may also be effective, especially as part of a long-term behavioural programme. Effective ways for the clinical management of physical withdrawal symptoms, both prophylactic (e.g. transient perioperative administration of methadone) and therapeutic (e.g. continuation of maintenance programs), are outlined in Table 11.5.

Transient perioperative administration of methadone

The time of last opioid exposure prior to hospital admission should be identified before commencing withdrawal prophylaxis with methadone.[31,39] Transient background therapy with methadone ensures the patient's optimal mental and physical stabilization. Methadone has a long half-life (mean 1.5 days) which permits once a day administration for a long-lasting preventive effect without toxic complications.[15,17]

Perioperative background therapy with methadone prevents withdrawal symptoms but without significant analgesic effect. Alternatively, other μ-agonist opioids such as morphine, sufentanil or fentanyl can be administered as an intravenous infusion to prevent withdrawal symptoms with hyperalgesia.[25a,38] The alpha-adrenoceptor agonist clonidine may reduce withdrawal symptoms and postoperative opioid demand, but its analgesic potency is lower compared with opioids.[40] In addition clonidine may induce sedation and physical inactivity, which may be undesirable during the early postoperative activation.

Continuation of opioid maintenance programmes

Patients should be commenced preoperatively on maintenance with methadone (the Methadone Maintenance Program; MMP)[21] or maintenance with buprenorphine[41] both of which should be continued as background therapy.[19] These patients need effective analgesia often with high

---

Table 11.5 Clinical management of physical withdrawal symptoms (prophylactic or therapeutic) in patients with opioid SUD

Administration of methadone*
(A) *Recovering patients enrolled in maintenance programs*
 Methadone racemate or levomethadone (in Germany)
 Daily dose at the same time as usual (oral or s.c./i.m.; relation oral to parenteral: 2:1)
 10 mg methadone racemate p.o. = 5 mg l-methadone p.o.
 5 mg methadone racemate s.c. = 2.5 mg l-methadone s.c.

(B) *SUD in patients not enrolled in maintenance programs*
 Methadone racemate   Levomethadone
 20–40 mg p.o. q24 h   10–20 mg p.o. q24 h
 10–20 mg s.c./i.m. q24 h   5–10 mg s.c./i.m. q24 h
 1.25–2.5 mg i.v. q5–10 min   0.06–1.25 mg i.v. q5–10 min
 (titrated injections to diminish or to avoid withdrawal symptoms)

Administration of other pure μ-opioid receptor agonists instead of methadone*
(intravenous infusion with morphine, fentanyl, hydromorphone)
Equianalgesic relations (s.c./i.m.): 10 mg morphine = 0.3 mg fentanyl = 1.5 mg
hydromorphone = 10 mg methadone racemat = 5 mg levomethadone

Administration of the α-2-adrenoceptor agonist clonidine (i.v., p.o.)

Administration of buprenorphine (only for patients enrolled in the maintenance program with buprenorphine)
• Sublingual: daily dose at the same time as usual
• s.c./i.m.: relation sublingual to parenteral: 2:1
 (in some countries the parenteral application of buprenorphine is not available: switching
 to methadone is advised (0.8 mg buprenorphine s.c./i.m. = 10 mg methadone racemat
 s.c./i.m. − 5 mg levo-methadone s.c./i.m. − 10 mg morphine s.c./i.m.)

Administration of naltrexone (p.o.)
• The optimum solution is to discontinue naltrexone 24–48 h prior to surgery, otherwise postoperative analgesic effectiveness of opioids is diminished and/or withdrawal symptoms may occur
• Careful titration of analgesic opioids is advised

---

i.v.: intravenous; p.o.: postoperatively; s.c.: subcutaneous; i.m.: intramuscularly.
*Methadone is indicated for prevention or therapy of withdrawal symptoms. The effective doses do not provide analgesia for acute pain.

---

doses of opioids. However, chronic opioid therapy, including methadone, can induce hyperalgesia and abnormal pain intensity, as well as cross tolerance.[23–25, 42,43] Thus, morphine as an opiod with a short half life rather than methadone is the opioid of choice for analgesia in patients enrolled in MMP. Doses of methadone high enough to provide pain relief may be dangerous.[29] In contrast buprenorphine should be used for analgesia as well as for backgound therapy in patients on a buprenorphine maintenance programme. If the analgesic control proves to be insufficient, switching from buprenorphine to methadone (substitution) plus morphine (analgesia) is recommended. Sublingual buprenorphine 0.4 mg is equivalent to oral racemic methadone 20 mg.[28] Background maintenance with methadone or buprenorphine should also be applied to patients underoging regional analgesic techniques.

Opioid antagonists.   Naloxone is an injectable, intravenous and short-acting antagonist. It should be avoided in opioid-dependent patients, otherwise hyperalgesia[44] with severe postoperative pain, and elevated systemic concentrations of catecholamines[20] with increased risk of cardiac complications may occur.[45,46] Naloxone titrated carefully against respiratory response should only be used for life-threatening toxic effects. If necessary this may be followed by a continuous intravenous infusion of naloxone at two-thirds of the initial intravenous dose per hour.[47]

Naltrexone is a long-acting and orally active opioid receptor antagonist. Long-term treatment with naltrexone may be indicated as an integral part of behavioural programs for patient rehabilitation. Naltrexone prevents the euphoric effects of opioid detoxification[21,48] as well as the psychological effects of alcohol.[49] Naltrexone inhibits the analgesic action of perioperatively administered μ-opioid receptor agonists and is associated with increased postoperative opioid requirement.[49] Furthermore, residual naltrexone activity may result in opioid withdrawal symptoms during analgesic opioid therapy (Table 11.5).[8,50,51] Naltrexone has a half-life of 3–4 h, and its active metabolite 6-naltrexone has a half-life of 9 h.[48] Therefore, naltrexone should be discontinued at least 24 h prior to surgery. Selective upregulation of μ-opioid receptors with increasing opioid sensitivity may develop and persist after discontinuation due to the previous blocking of μ-opioid receptors with naltrexone.[52] Postoperative opioids should be titrated carefully.

Alcohol

Organ damage is common and is associated with an increased risk of postoperative complications.[31,32,53] Psychological dependence, tolerance, physical dependence and psychiatric disorders are often severe.[54,55] As with opioid withdrawal the symptoms of alcohol withdrawal can be quantified using a simple scoring system, the revised Clinical Institute Withdrawal Assessment of Alcohol (CIWA-Ar) scale.[56] Withdrawal seizures and delirium can be life-threatening. Thus, the prevention of withdrawal symptoms perioperatively is important.[56–60] Alcoholics exhibit neuronal hyperexcitability which has been shown to increase during clinical or experimental withdrawal.[11,55] The increased neuronal hyperexcitability results in difficult pain control requiring high doses of opioids in the postoperative period, although there is no cross tolerance between alcohol and opioids.[15] In order to improve the pulmonary, cardiac and gastrointestinal functions effective analgesia is as important as in other patients without SUD.[37]

Advice on choice of anaesthesia is given in Table 11.3. Peripheral alcoholic polyneuropathy can be associated with sympathetic dysregulations (hypotonia) and reduced efficacy of local anaesthetics. Analgesic therapy can be difficult and the whole spectrum of multimodal analgesia should be used (Table 11.4).[61]

Withdrawal prophylaxis and treatment

Cross tolerance between alcohol and benzodiazepines[15] means that it is possible to accomplish both prevention and treatment of alcohol withdrawal symptoms by substituting a long-acting benzodiazepine such as flunitrazepam. Adjuvant drugs such as clonidine and beta-blockers are recommended to reduce the intense sympathetic stimulation, and haloperidol to diminish hallucinations.[40,58–60]

Although prophylactic intravenous infusion of low doses of ethyl alcohol may be effective, recent evidence-based guidelines do not support this practice.[58] Clonidine and neuroleptic agents may decrease the seizure threshold, but should only be co-administered with to benzodiazepines.[58] Low potency aliphatic phenothiazines, such as chlorpromazine, or thioxanthenes, such as chlorprothixene, diminish the seizure threshold more than other neuroleptics.[62] Withdrawal prophylaxis and withdrawal therapy with clonidine, benzodiazepines and clomethiazol, should be tapered slowly over days (clonidine) to weeks (benzodiazepines) to prevent withdrawal symptoms for the substituted substances.

Volatile nitrates, solvents and fuels

There is an enormous variety of solvents and fuels that are used, including almost any household cleaning agent or propellant, paint thinner, glue and lighter fluid. Children and teenagers are more likely to abuse solvents than other CNS-depressant substances. Solvents produce euphoria and other effects similar to subanaesthetic concentrations of volatile anaesthetics as well as CNS depression similar to alcohol intoxication. Physical dependence is rare but psychological dependence and tolerance can develop.[33] Acute effects include asphyxia, sudden sniffing death syndrome, and serious injury due to falls, burns, etc. Chronic inhalant abuse can cause cardiovascular and respiratory depression and the interaction with halogenated hydrocarbons may induce life-threatening dysrhythmias. Solvent abuse can also damage renal, hepatic and neurological systems. Diagnosis of inhalant abuse is particularly difficult, relying almost entirely on a thorough history and a high index of suspicion. No specific laboratory tests confirm solvent inhalation.[63,64]

Benzodiazepines and barbiturates

Polysubstance abusers prefer long-acting benzodiazepines such as flunitrazepam or diazepam, or even barbiturates for self-treatment of withdrawal symptoms due to alcohol or opioids.[15,31,34,39,65] Isolated SUD with low dosages of benzodiazepines is also reported.[66] Advice on choice of anaesthesia is given in Table 11.3. Initial analgesic opioid dosages are the same as in patients without SUD, however, increasing dosages of μ-agonist opioids should be titrated carefully since there is no cross tolerance to opioids.[15] The whole spectrum of multimodal analgesia should be used (Table 11.4).[63]

SUD with CNS-stimulant Substances

Cocaine and amphetamines

Cocaine, crack cocaine, amphetamines and amphetamine-like designer drugs such as ecstasy are psychostimulants with potential for toxic activity.[15] Amphetamines are prescribed as anorectics or stimulants against fatigue, whereas all the others are illicit drugs.

The extent of pre-existing organ damage and substance-induced mental disorders may be severe (Table 11.2).[32] After exposure to cocaine and crack cocaine intensive stimulating psychotropic and sympathetic cardiovascular effects are observed, which afterwards are followed by predominantly affective withdrawal symptoms associated with craving behaviour, exhaustion, dysphoria, depression, anxiety, and finally fatigue with a strong desire for sleep.[5,11,14,15] The intensive sympathetic stimulation can be life-threatening.[14] Mental disturbances are sometimes difficult to distinguish from acute substance effects or psychological withdrawal symptoms. Thus, the observation of physiological signs of acute substance effects (mydriasis, tachycardia and hypertension) may be helpful.[14]

Advice on choice of anaesthesia is given in Table 11.3. Anaesthesia is dangerous during acute exposure to cocaine or other excitatory drugs and should be avoided until the acute effects have disappeared. Initial analgesic opioid dosages are the same as in patients without SUD, but increasing dosages of μ-agonists should be titrated carefully due to the lack of cross tolerance to opioids.[67] Diminished aggregation of thrombocytes may occur in some patients with cocaine dependence.

Severe mental disturbance often results in these patients having an increased analgesic requirement (Table 11.4). Psychic/psychological withdrawal symptoms should be treated symptomatically.

Cannabis (marijuana)

Marijuana is the most commonly used illegal drug in the US and many other countries. The major drug of the cannabinoids is delta-9-tetrahydrocannabinol (THC). Marijuana is usually smoked, whereas intravenous injections are rare. Orthostatic disturbances as well as hyperthermia[68] may occur during exposure to cannabinoids. Patients with frequent cannabis abuse tend to suffer from chronic obstructive pulmonary changes and pulmonary infections.

Advice on choice of anaesthesia is given in Table 11.3. Anaesthesia during acute exposure with excitatory drugs is dangerous and should be avoided until the acute effects have disappeared. There are no special analgesic considerations (Table 11.4); because of the lack of physical withdrawal symptoms[69] monitoring and symptomatic treatment of mental disturbances take priority.

Lysergic acid diethylamine and phencyclidine

Psychedelic agents induce hallucinations, illusions and disordered thought processes. The hallucinogenic substances lysergic acid diethylamine (LSD), phencyclidine (PCP) and 3,4-methylenedioxymethamphetamine (MDMA; ecstacy) are the most common illicit psychedelic drugs.[30] Chronic use of LSD is frequently associated with persistent psychiatric disorders.[31] A small proportion of former LSD users describe episodic visual disturbances, flashes of colour, pseudo-hallucinations, and remembering of prior experiences with LSD (flash back).[69]

Advice on choice of anaesthesia is given in Table 11.3. Anaesthesia during acute exposure with excitatory drugs is dangerous and should be avoided until acute effects have disappeared. There are no special analgesic considerations with sole LSD use (Table 11.4). Cross tolerance to opioids is unknown.[69]

Patients in Drug-free Recovery

It is self-evident that these patients have a past history of addiction. But being in drug-free recovery means more than just abstinence from psychotropic drugs. These patients have successfully undergone withdrawal from opioids or other drugs, and are trying to keep their propensity for addiction under control. Often former addicts who are drug abstinent will be participating in personal recovery programs, such as the 12-step fellowship programs, or may be involved in support groups such as

Alcoholics Anonymous or Narcotics Anonymous. Furthermore, many former addicts will be involved in drug rehabilitation programmes such as opioid agonist therapy (viz. substitution with methadone or buprenorphine), or opioid antagonist (naltrexone) therapy.

The development of hyperalgesia has been described after experimental opioid abstinence.[70] After therapeutic detoxification of opioids a persistent and significant autonomic nervous system instability, diminished pain tolerance, increased pain intensity and increased sensitivity to exogenous opioids have been observed over several months (protracted abstinence syndrome).[67,71,72] These patients require careful titration of analgesic opioids in order to avoid accidental and life-threatening side effects. The duration of protracted abstinence syndrome is unknown.

Anaesthesia

The extent of organic and psychiatric illness should be estimated in the same manner as in any other patient. Long-acting opioids are undesirable because of psychotropic effects following awakening and should be avoided. Short-acting opioids (e.g. alfentanil and sufentanil) can be used safely during anaesthesia. However, acute tolerance and hyperalgesia has been described after use of the ultra short-acting opioid remifentanil.[73–75] This phenomenon is as counter productive in patients with active SUD as in non-addicted patients. Other µ-opioid agonists should be preferred. Non-opioid analgesics can be used as premedicants or shortly before the end of anaesthesia, together with local anaesthetics (nerve blocks, subcutaneous infiltration and catheter techniques).[26]

Analgesia

Patients in drug-free recovery are often anxious not to become 're-addicted' subsequent to medical administration of psychoactive drugs (opioids, sedatives, etc.). Several processes of neuronal plasticity in the CNS may induce long-lasting sensitivity and memory concerning psychotropic drug effects.[3–5] Patients with a history of SUD show a high incidence of anxiety and mental instability under stressful situations such as trauma and surgery, making them more vulnerable to any kind of stress and pain than patients without SUD.[76] It has become obvious that analgesic undertreatment plays an important role in pseudoaddictive behaviour[77] and may provoke relapse into SUD.[12,78] This requires effective psychological support by health care professionals and family members, and most importantly effective analgesic treatment. SUD patients need

Table 11.6 Points to consider in the perioperative anaesthetic and analgesic management of patients in drug-free recovery

- Evaluate the extent of recovery (drugs during active addiction, abstinence, time course, involvement in recovery programs, history of relapse(s), social circumstances, maintenance program)
- Estimate pre-existing organic diseases and psychological alterations
- Clarify the expected intensity of nociceptive stimulation by surgery
  - Advise prior to surgery about possibilities of effective postoperative analgesia. Be aware of two problems: patients' fear of relapse due to psychotropic opioid effects, and the possibility relapse due to analgesic undertreatment
- Involve family members or important contact persons, also an addiction specialist
- Organize an individual anaesthetic and analgesic plan including special care by an Acute Pain Service
- Manage postoperative pain relief by means of non-opioids first, gradually adapt mild or strong opioids to avoid analgesic undertreatment
- Prefer regional catheter techniques, other regional analgesia methods, non-opioid drugs and other non-pharmacological procedures (acupuncture, TENS, physical therapy)
- Use strong opioids as part of multimodal analgesia if necessary, but titrate very carefully to avoid psychotropic effects (intravenous PCA, oral sustained release formulations, rectal)
- Avoid prescription of any centrally acting drug without the patient's agreement
- Supervise discharge medications and activate recovery program

effective analgesia just the same as other patients in order to improve postoperative functional outcome.[37]

The whole spectrum of postoperative analgesia regimens, including strong opioids if necessary should be considered. Postoperative analgesia should be discussed as early as possible with the patient, his family, the sponsor and others. Adequate and stepwise-adapted analgesia is necessary. Analgesic management will depend on the type of surgery but will need to take into account a number of important points as outlined in Table 11.6.

Minor and moderate surgery
All forms of non-opioid pain regimens (NSAID, paracetamol, antispasmodics, dipyrone, clonidine, physical therapy, transcutaneous electrical nerve simulation (TENS), acupuncture and regional analgesia with local anesthetics) can be used. If non-opioid analgesia is ineffective, the mild opioid tramadol, which is non-scheduled, can be administered.[79–81] About 10% of patients cannot metabolize tramadol to its analgesically active metabolite (non-responders).[82] Alternatively, the partial agonist buprenorphine with its low addiction potential may be used, but its ceiling effect may prevent effective titrated analgesia.[26] Alternatively, strong μ-agonist opioids may be used in conjunction with non-opioid analgesics as multimodal analgesia, if previous analgesic steps proved to be ineffective. Initial dosages should be as low as possible and titrated to effective pain relief.

Major surgery

Following major surgery all patients with SUD need highly effective analgesia (intravenous PCA, regional analgesia) in the same way as any other patient.[83] The use of low doses of morphine by intravenous PCA with optimum control of any opioid effects[76] while avoiding high concentrations in the brain,[84,85] may be an important alternative technique to regional catheters. These could reactivate the addiction memory[3–5] with subsequent relapse. Non-opioids should be used as much as possible. As with subcutaneous PCA in patients without SUD,[86] repeated subcutaneous injections of low doses (5 mg) of morphine are an effective option.

Summary

The special problems of postoperative analgesia in patients with SUD are described. SUD with one substance only is becoming less common while the number of polysubstance abusers is increasing. Patients with SUD may have multiple organic diseases, impaired immune response and substance-induced disorders (intoxication, withdrawal, psychiatric and behavioural abnormalities), often associated with low compliance and craving behaviour.

The perioperative management should focus on four problems:

- prevention of physical withdrawal symptoms in patients with SUD using CNS-depressant substances;
- symptomatic treatment of affective withdrawal symptoms in patients suffering from SUD with CNS-stimulant substances;
- anaesthesia (regional or general-plus-regional) which takes into consideration the different organic diseases;
- postoperative multimodal analgesia (non-opioids plus opioids) with a preference for regional analgesia techniques.

Patients enrolled in preoperative maintenance programs (methadone and buprenorphine) need their daily maintenance opioid dosage as baseline. This baseline therapy does not, however, provide analgesia. Therefore, these patients need in addition a short-acting opioid, often at a higher dose than usual but which, due to opioid tolerance, does not cause respiratory depression. Conversely, use of regional analgesia in patients enrolled on maintenance programs should not result in withdrawal of prophylaxis; these patients need maintenance opioid. Patients with a past history of SUD have both an intense fear of relapsing into active SUD and a fear of suffering from postoperative pain. These patients require anaesthesia and analgesia adapted to the type of surgery and pain intensity. Withholding effective analgesic treatment can paradoxically lead to relapse in SUD recovered patients. Furthermore, the commonly held opinion by health care providers that it is desirable to withhold strong opioids from SUD recovered patients is obsolete. However, in order to avoid psychotropic effects the dosages of opioids as well as the analgesic effectiveness should be monitored closely.

References

1. Working Group on the Misuse of Alcohol and Drugs by Doctors. London: British Medical Association, 1998.
2. DSM IV. Diagnostic and Statistical Manual of Mental Disorders, 4th ed. Washington, DC: American Psychiatric Association, 1994.
3. Jasinski DR. Assessment of the abuse potentiality of morphine like drugs (methods used in man). In: Martin WR (ed.) Drug Addiction I. Handbook of Experimental Pharmacology, vol. 45/I. New York: Springer-Verlag, 1977; 197–258.
4. Cami J, Farré M. Drug addiction. New Engl J Med 2003; 349: 975–986.
5. Nestler EJ. Molecular basis of long-term plasticity underlying addiction. Nature Rev Neurosci 2001; 2: 119–128.
6. Savage SR, Joranson DE, Covingston EC, Schnoll SH, Heit HA, Gilson AM. Definitions related to the medical use of opioids: evolution towards universal agreement. J Pain Sympt Manage 2003; 26: 655–667.
7. Balster RL. Neural basis of inhalant abuse. Drug Alcohol Depend 1998; 51: 207–214.
8. Kessler RC, McGonagle KA, Zaho S et al. Lifetime and 12-month prevalance of DSM-III-R psychiatric disorders in the United States. Arch Gen Psych 1994; 51: 8–19.
9. Anthony JC, Helzer JE. Syndromes of drug abuse and dependence. In: Robins LN, Regier DA (eds) Psychiatric Disorders in America: The Epidemiologic Catchment Area Study. New York: The Free Press, Mac Millan Inc., 1991; 116–154.
10. Caumo W, Schmidt AP, Schneider CN et al. Preoperative predictors of moderate to intense acute postoperative pain in patients undergoing abdominal surgery. Acta Anaesthesiol Scand 2002; 46: 1265–1271.
11. Compton P, Gebhardt GF. The neurophysiology of pain in addiction. In: Graham AW, Schultz TK (eds) Principles of Addiction Medicine, 2nd ed. Chevy Chase, Maryland: American Society of Addiction Medicine, 1998; 901–917.
12. Savage SR. Addiction in the treatment of pain: significance, recognition and treatment. Pain Sympt Manage 1993; 8: 265–278.
13. Cone EJ, Fant RV, Rohay JM et al. Oxycodone involvement in drug abuse deaths: a DAWN-based classification scheme applied to an oxycodone postmortem database containing over 1000 cases. J Analyt Toxicol 2003; 27: 57–67.
14. Mendelsohn JH, Mello NK. Management of cocaine abuse and dependence. New Engl J Med 1996; 334: 965–972.
15. Jaffe JH. Drug addiction and drug abuse. In: Gilman AG, Rall TW, Nies AS, Taylor P (eds) Goodman and Gilman's the Pharmacological Basis of Therapeutics, 8th ed. New York: Pergamon Press, 1990; 522–573.

16. Stimmel B. Pain and its Relief without Addiction. Clinical Issues in the Use of Opioids and Other Analgesics. New York: The Haworth Medical Press, Inc., 1997.

17. Kreek MJ, Koob GF. Drug Dependence: Stress and Dysregulation of Brain Reward Pathways. Drug Alcohol Depend 1998; 51: 23–47.

18. Martin WR, Sloan JW. Morphine dependence. In: Martin WR (ed.) Drug Addiction I. Handbook of Experimental Pharmacology, vol. 45/I. New York: Springer-Verlag, 1977; 43–158.

19. Beattie Ch, Mark L, Umbricht-Schneiter A. Evaluation of the patient with alcoholism and other dependencies. In: Longnecker DE, Tinker JH, Morgan Jr GE (eds) Principles and Practice of Anesthesiology, 2nd ed. St Louis: Mosby, 1998; 537–565.

20. Kienbaum P, Thürauf N, Michel MS *et al*. Profound increase in epinephrine concentration in plasma and cardiovascular stimulation after mu-opioid receptor blockade in opioid-addicted patients during barbiturate-induced anesthesia for acute detoxification. Anesthesiology 1998; 88: 1154–1161.

21. Kreek MJ. Long-term pharmacotherapy for opiate (primarily heroin) addiction: opioid agonists. In: Schuster CR, Kuhar MJ (eds) Pharmacological Aspects of Drug Dependence. Toward an Integrated Neurobehavioral Approach. Handbook of Experimental Pharmacology, vol. 118. Berlin: Springer-Verlag, 1996; 487–562.

22. Cox BM. Mechanisms of tolerance. In: Stein Ch (ed.) Opioids in Pain Control. Basis and Clinical Aspects. Cambridge: Cambridge University Press, 1999; 109–130.

23. Doverty M, White JM, Somogyi AA *et al*. Hyperalgesic responses in methadone maintenance patients. Pain 2001; 90: 91–96.

24. Mao J. Opioid-induced abnormal pain sensibility: implications in clinical opioid therapy. Pain 2002; 100: 213–217.

25. Ballantyne JC, Mao J. Opioid therapy for chronic pain. New Engl J Med 2003; 349: 1943–1953.

26. Jage J, Bey T. Postoperative analgesia in patients with substance use disorders: Part I. Acute Pain 2000; 3: 140–155.

27. Jage J, Bey T. Postoperative analgesia in patients with substance use disorders: Part II. Acute Pain 2000; 3: 172–180.

27a. Mitra S, Sinatra RS. Perioperative management of acute pain in the opioid-dependent patient. Anesthesiology 2004; 101: 212–227.

28. Foley KM. Opiod analgesics in clinical management. In: Herz A (ed) Opiods II. Handbook of Experimental Pharmacology, vol. 104/II. New York: Springer-Verlag, 1993; 697–743.

29. Walker PW, Klein D, Kasza L. High methadone and ventricular arrhythmias: a report of three cases. Pain 2003; 103: 321–324.

30. Steindler EM. ASAM addiciton terminology. In: Graham AW, Schultz TK (eds) Principles of Addiction Medicine, 2nd ed. Chevy Chase, Maryland: American Society of Addiction Medicine, Inc., 1998; 1301 1304.

31. Caldwell III TB. Anesthesia for patients with behavioral and environmental disorders. In: Katz J, Benumof JL, Kadis LB (eds) Anesthesia and Uncommon Diseases, 3rd ed. Philadelphia: WB Saunders, 1990; 792–922.

32. Cisek JE. Substance users. In: Goldfrank LR, Flomenbaum NE, Lewin NA, Weisman RS, Howland MA, Hoffman RS (eds) Goldfrank's Toxicologic Emergencies, 6th ed. Stanford, Connecticut: Appleton & Lange, 1998; 1729–1740.

33. Wood PR, Soni N. Anaesthesia and substance abuse. Anaesthesia 1989, 44: 672–680.
34. Jage J. Anaesthesia and analgesia in opiate dependence. Anaesthesist 1988; 37: 470–482.
35. Latasch I, Christ R. Anaesthetic problems in drug addicts. Anaesthesist 1988; 37: 123–139.
36. Brodner G, Mertes N, Buerkle H et al. Acute pain management: analysis, implications and consequences after prospective experience with 6349 surgical patients. Eur J Anaesth 2000; 17: 566–575.
37. Kehlet H, Wilmore DW. Multimodal strategies to improve surgical outcome. Am J Surg 2002; 183: 630–641.
38. Bradley BP, Gossop M, Phillips GT, Legarda JJ. The development of an opiate withdrawal scale (OWS). Br J Addict 1987; 82: 1139–1142.
39. McCammon RL. Anesthesia for the chemically dependent patient. In: Review Course Lectures 1986. Cleveland, Ohio: IARS, 1986; 47–55.
40. Maze M, Tranquili W. Alpha2-adrenoceptor agonists: defining the role in clinical anesthesia. Anesthesiology 1991; 74: 581–605.
41. Johnson RE, Jaffe JH, Fudala PJ. A controlled trial of buprenorphine treatment for opioid dependence. J Am Med Assoc 1992; 287: 2750–2755.
42. Doverty M, Somogyi AA, White JM et al. Methadone maintenance patients are cross-tolerant to the antinociceptive effects of morphine. Pain 2001; 93: 155–163.
43. Mercadante S, Ferrera P, Villari P, Arcuri E. Hyperalgesia: an emerging iatrogenic syndrome. J Pain Sympt Manage 2003; 26: 769–775.
44. Bederson J, Field H, Barbaro N. Hyperalgesia during naloxone precipitated withdrawal from morphine is associated with increased on-cell activity in the rostral ventromedial medulla. Somatosens Motor Res 1990; 2: 185–188.
45. Andree RA. Sudden death following naloxone administration. Anesth Analg 1980; 59: 782–784.
46. Levin ER, Sharp B, Drayer JIM, Weber MA. Severe hypertension induced by naloxone. Am J Med Sci 1985; 290: 70–72.
47. Manfredi PL, Ribeiro S, Cahndler SW, Payne R. Inappropriate use of naloxone in cancer patients with pain. J Pain Sympt Manage 1996; 11: 131–134.
48. Gonzales JP, Brogden RN. Naltrexone: a review of its pharmacodynamic and pharmacokinetic properties and therapeutic efficacy in the treatment of opioid dependence. Drugs 1988; 35: 192–213.
49. Volpicelli JR, Alterman AI, Hayashida M, O'Brian CP. Naltrexone in the treatment of alcohol dependence. Arch Gen Psychiatr 1992; 49: 876–880.
50. American Hospital Formulary Service (AHFS). Bethesda, Maryland: American Society of Health-System Pharmacists, Inc., 1999; 1839–1846.
51. Loimer N, Linzmayer L, Grünberger J. Comparison between observer assessment and self rating of withdrawal distress during opiate detoxification. Drug Alcohol Depend 1991; 28: 265–268.
52. Millan MJ, Morris BJ, Herz A. Antagonist-induced opioid receptor up-regulation: characterization of supersensitivity to selective mu and delta agonists. J Pharmacol Exp Ther 1988; 247: 721–727.
53. Tsueda K, Lloyd GE, Heine MF et al. Opiates in ethanol withdrawal. Anesth Analg 1995; 81: 874–877.
54. Bruce DL. Alcoholism and anesthesia. Anesth Analg 1983; 62: 84–89.
55. Samson HH, Harris RA. Neurobiology of alcohol abuse. TIPS 1992; 13: 206–211.

56. Sullivan JT, Sykora K, Schneiderman J *et al*. Assessment of alcohol withdrawal: the revised clinical institute withdrawal assessment of alcohol scale (CIWA-Ar). Br J Addict 1989; 84: 1353–1357.

57. Tabakoff B, Hellevuo K, Hoffman PL. Alcohol. In: Schuster CR, Kuhar MJ (eds) Pharmacological Aspects of Drug Dependence. Toward an Integrated Neurobehavioral Approach. Handbook of Experimental Pharmacology, vol. 118. Berlin: Springer-Verlag, 1996; 373–458.

58. Mayo-Smith MF for the American Society of Addiction Medicine Working Group on pharmacological management of alcohol withdrawal. Jr Am Med Assoc 1997; 278: 144–151.

59. Spiess CD, Rommelspacher H. Alcohol withdrawal in the surgical patient: prevention and treatment. Anesth Analg 1999; 88: 946–954.

60. The Plinius Major Society. Guidelines on evaluation of treatment of alcohol dependence. Alcoholism 1994; 30(Suppl): 1–8.

61. Kehlet H, Dahl JB. The value of 'multimodal' or 'balanced analgesia' in postoperative pain treatment. Anesth Analg 1993; 77: 1048–1056.

62. Baldessarini RJ. Drugs and the treatment of psychiatric disorders. In: Hardman JG, Limbird LE, Molinoff PB, Ruddon RW, Gilman AG (eds) Goodman and Gilman's the Pharmacological Basis of Therapeutics, 9th ed. New York: Pergamon Press, 1996; 399–430.

63. Brouette T, Anton R. Clinical review of inhalants. Am J Addict 2001; 10: 79–94.

64. Anderson CE, Loomis GA. Recognition and prevention of inhalant abuse. Am Fam Physician 2003; 68: 869–874.

65. Eickelberg SJ, Mayo-Smith M. Management of sedative-hypnotic intoxication and withdrawal. In: Graham AW, Schultz TK (eds) Principles of Addiction Medicine, 2nd ed. Chevy Chase, Maryland: American Society of Addition Medicine, Inc., 1998; 441–455.

66. Owen RT, Tyrer P. Benzodiazepine dependence. Drugs 1983; 25: 385–398.

67. O'Brien CP. Drug addiction and drug abuse. In: Hardman JG, Limbird LE, Molinoff PB, Ruddon RW, Gilman AG (eds) Goodman and Gilman's. The Pharmacological Basis of Therapeutics, 9th ed. New York: Pergamon Press, 1996; 557–577.

68. Walter FG, Bey TA, Ruschke DS *et al*. Marihuana and hyperthermia. J Toxicol Clin Toxicol 1996; 34: 217–221.

69. Wilkins JN, Conner BT, Gorelick DA. Management of stimulant, hallucinogen, marijuana and phencyclidine intoxications and withdrawal. In: Graham AW, Schultz TK (eds) Principles of Addiction Medicine, 2nd ed. Chevy Chase, Maryland: American Society of Addiction Medicine, Inc., 1998; 465–485.

70. Li X, Clark JD. Hyperalgesia during opioid abstinence: mediation by glutamate and substance P. Anesth Analg 2002; 95: 979–984.

71. Martin WR, Jasinski DR. Physiological parameters of morphine dependence in man tolerance, early abstinence, protracted abstinence. J Psychiatr Res 1969; 7: 9–17.

72. Strang J, McCambridge J, Best D *et al*. Loss of tolerance and overdose mortality after inpatient opiate detoxification: follow up study. Br Med J 2003; 326: 959–960.

73. Guignard B, Bossard AE, Coste C *et al*. Acute tolerance. Intraoperative remifentanil increases postoperative pain and morphine requirement. Anesthesiology 2000; 93: 409–417.

74. Koppert W, Sittl R, Scheubner K *et al*. Differential modulation of remifentanil-induced analgesia and postinfusion hyperalgesia by S-ketamine and clonidine in humans. Anesthesiology 2003; 99: 152–159.

75. Angst MS, Koppert W, Pahl I et al. Short-term infusion of the mu-opioid agonist remifentanil in humans causes hyperalgesia during withdrawal. Pain 2003; 106: 49–57.
76. Beattie C, Umbricht-Schneiter A, Mark L. Anesthesia and analgesia. In: Graham AW, Schultz TK (eds) Principles of Addiction Medicine, 2nd ed. Chevy Chase, Maryland: American Society of Addiction Medicine, Inc., 1998; 877–889.
77. Weissman DE, Haddox DE. Opioid pseudoaddiction: an iatrogenic syndrome. Pain 1989; 36: 363–366.
78. Passik SD, Portenoy RK. Substance abuse issues. In: Ashburn MA, Rice LJ (eds) The Management of Pain. New York: Churchill Livingstone, 1998; 51–61.
79. Stamer UM, Maier C, Grind S et al. Tramadol in the management of post-operative pain: a double blind, placebo- and active drug-controlled study. Eur J Anaesthesiol 1997; 14: 646–654.
80. Scott LJ, Perry CM. Tramadol. A review of its use in perioperative pain. Drugs 2000; 60: 139–176.
81. Murano T, Yamamoto H, Endo N et al. Studies of dependence on tramadol in rats. Arzneimittel-Forsch./Drug Res 1978; 28: 152–158.
82. Stamer UM, Lehnen K, Hothker F et al. Impact of CYP2D6 genotype on postoperative tramadol analgesia. Pain 2003; 105: 231–238.
83. Kehlet H, Holte K. Effect of postoperative analgesia on surgical outcome. Br J Anaesth 2001; 87: 62–72.
84. Oldendorf WH, Hyman S, Braun L, Oldendorf SZ. Blood–brain barrier: penetration of morphine, codeine, heroin, and methadone after carotidic injection. Science 1972; 178: 984–985.
85. von Cube B, Teschemacher Hj, Herz A, Hess R. Permeation of morphine-like acting substances to their sites of antinociceptive action in the brain after intravenous and intraventricular application and dependence upon lipid-solubility. Naunyn-Schmiedebergs Arch Pharmakol 1970; 265: 455–473.
86. Doyle E, Morton NS, McNicol LR. Comparison of patient-controlled analgesia in children by i.v. and s.c. routes of administration. Br J Anaesth 1994; 72: 533–536.

Appendix: SUD-related definitions

Addiction   Commonly used term meaning the aberrant use of a specific psychoactive substance in a manner characterized by loss of control, compulsive use, preoccupation and continued use despite harm; pejorative term, replaced in the DSM-IV in a non-pejorative way by the term SUD with psychological and physical dependence.

Dependence
Psychological dependence: need for a specific psychoactive substance either for its positive effects or to avoid negative psychological/physical effects associated with its withdrawal.

Physical dependence: a physiological state of adaptation to a specific psychoactive substance characterized by the emergence of a withdrawal syndrome during abstinence, which may be relieved in total or in part by readministration of the substance.

Chemical dependence A generic term relating to psychological and/or physical dependence on one or more psychoactive substances (11 classes of psychoactive substances are abused: alcohol; sedatives, hypnotics and anxiolytics; cannabis; opioids; cocaine; amphetamine and other sympathomimetics; hallucinogens; inhalants; caffeine; nicotine; PCP).

Substance use disorders Term of DSM-IV comprising two main groups: Substance dependence disorder and Substance-induced disorder, for example intoxication, withdrawal, delirium, psychotic disorders

Tolerance A state in which an increased dosage of a psychoactive substance is needed to produce a desired effect.

Cross tolerance: tolerance induced by repeated administration of one psychoactive substance that is manifested toward another substance to which the individual has not been recently exposed. Opioids induce typical side effects of sedation, cognitive impairment, nausea, or ventilatory depression. Tolerance to these effects develops within days or weeks, but almost never to analgesia or to constipation.

Withdrawal syndrome The onset of a predictable constellation of signs and symptoms following the abrupt discontinuation of or rapid decrease in dosage of a psychoactive substance.

Polydrug dependence Concomitant use of two or more psychoactive substances in quantities and frequencies that cause individually significant physiological, psychological and/or sociological distress or impairment (polysubstance abuser).

Recovery A process of overcoming both physical and psychological dependence on a psychoactive substance with a commitment to sobriety.

Abstinence Non-use of any psychoactive substance, in recovery.

Maintenance Prevention of craving behaviour and withdrawal symptoms of opioids by long-acting opioids (e.g. methadone and buprenorphine).

Substance abuse Use of a psychoactive substances in a manner outside of sociocultural conventions; according to this, any use of illicit and licit drugs in a manner not dictated by convention (e.g. according to physician's order) is abuse.

Index

Note: Numbers in **bold** refer to Figures and Tables.